Secrets
of The
Mommyhood

By Heather Alexander

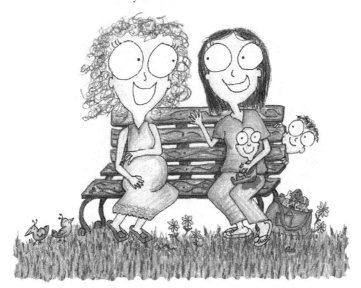

SPRIGGS
MERRIWETHER

Published by Spriggs Merriwether, LLC
Knoxville, TN 37922
©2012 Heather Alexander

Publisher's Cataloging-in-Publication Data

Alexander, Heather.
    Secrets of the mommyhood : everything I wish someone had told me
about pregnancy, childbirth and having a baby / Heather Alexander.
        p. cm.
    ISBN: 978-0-9850060-3-7
    1. Pregnancy—Popular works. 2. Childbirth—Popular works. 3.
Motherhood—Humor.   I. Title.
    RG525 .A515 2012
    618.2—dc23

                                                        2012906860

Editor: Heather Hopp-Bruce
Cover and interior design: Heather Hopp-Bruce
Illustrations: Heather Hopp-Bruce
Author photo: Photography by Sabrina

ISBN: 978-0-9850060-3-7
ISBN: 978-0-9850060-4-4 (eBook)
Library of Congress Control Number: 2012906860

PRINTED IN THE UNITED STATES OF AMERICA
10 9 8 7 6 5 4 3 2 1

SPRIGGS MERRIWETHER

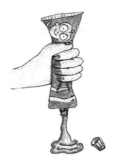

To all the moms in my life,
especially Paula Drake,
whose pregnancy inspired this book.

And to Molly and Charlie,
who taught me what it is to be a mom.

B efore I had kids, I thought if I read a million pregnancy and parenting books, I would be prepared
for everything motherhood could throw at me.
WRONG! Once I had kids, I often found myself with a
bubble over my head that read, "Why in the world didn't
someone tell me THAT?"

A couple of years later, I was invited to a baby shower
for a friend and wanted to include a funny note about
things that were coming her way – some advice based on
my Mommyhood experience. I kept it to ten things. But
my mind was swimming with so many more that I realized there were far more experiences to share.

I went to sleep. My five-and-a-half month-old woke
up just before 5:00 a.m. and, after feeding him, my mind
began to race with all the things I was failing to tell my
friend. Thus, the idea for this book was born.

Secrets of the Mommyhood is a light-hearted, real and
practical perspective on what really happens in the
trenches of motherhood. Those other books don't talk
nearly enough about poop, vomit and what's on TV at
3:00 a.m.!

I have a son and daughter and have been a working
mom and a stay-at-home mom. Do I have motherhood
all figured out? Absolutely not, but I can share with you
a few insights about what might happen and, hopefully,
make you laugh about it.

I am originally from Tennessee, but I also have lived in
Atlanta, Georgia, and Washington, D.C., where I worked
as a desk jockey for UPS. And for a few months at Christ-
mastime, I even drove a UPS delivery truck in the Metro
D.C. area to "learn the business." Yes, I was chased by
dogs, but even being chased by dogs couldn't prepare

me for what happened when I became a mom. So, here it is: the book I wish I had read before I had kids. I hope it helps you anticipate – with humor – some of the things that are coming your way.

Welcome to the Mommyhood!

Heather

A quick disclaimer

I am not a doctor (medical or Ph.D.). Almost everything in this book is based on personal experience. These are things about becoming a mom I learned along the way that I find funny, interesting or helpful. Advice given is not intended to replace the opinion of your personal physician or your child's pediatrician or your own best judgment.

Additionally, as of this writing, I am not affiliated in any way with individuals or companies who make products mentioned in this book.

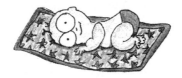

Table of Contents

CHAPTER FOUR
Assembling Your Babycare Team

CHAPTER FIVE
Childbirth

CHAPTER SIX
Newborns

CHAPTER ONE

The Original List That Started It All

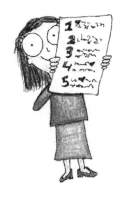

Ten Things No One Told Me Before I Had a Baby

1 **You can never** have enough pacifiers. Put more than one in each car, in your purse, etc. Somehow you never have one when you need it. And at some point, you will find the nearest grocery store and in desperation give your child one that hasn't been sterilized. This brings me to #2:

2 **Don't judge** other parents; it may be you one day. I remember having opinions about some harried mother with her ketchup-smothered child and thinking I would never be out and about with a ragamuffin. Been there. Same goes for a frustrated parent at the store who says something to their child that you find appalling. Been there, too.

3 **You will obsess** about your newborn's pee and poop. You and your husband will have entire conversations about its smell, consistency and regularity (or lack thereof) like it's the weather.

4 **Projectile vomit** and explosive poop is rare but real. If you leave the house without a change of clothes for your baby, you are actually throwing down a poop gauntlet.

5 **The surest way** to make your child pee, poop or spit up is to give them a bath.

6 **The second surest way** to make your child pee, poop or spit up is to take them to a photography session. I recommend a decoy outfit.

7 **Newborn babies** chortle and make many different noises when they sleep. It's really hard for you to fall asleep when they are making those noises. Then when things are too quiet, you also can't sleep. Your new mommy eyes become catlike and you can almost see in the dark as you check to make sure your baby's chest is going up and down.

8 **Total strangers** will touch your baby's face and worse – their hands. Those hands go right in the mouth. You also will look at other people's kids and see microscopic germs swirling around them like an aura. In crowded spaces, I recommend putting a blanket over the carrier or closing it up so people won't be tempted to touch your baby.

9 **Passing around a baby** that has just been fed is like shaking up a can of soda and then opening it. Most new parents learn this lesson the hard way.

10 **When you are pregnant** and hands-free, everyone will hold the door open for you. When you are pushing a stroller and could really use some help with the door, it won't occur to anyone (except another mom) to help you.

CHAPTER TWO

Expectantly
Expecting

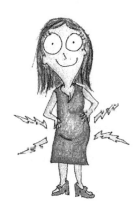

The Bump Watch

This time it's you. Not your friend, not your cousin, not so-and-so from work…YOU are pregnant. Congratulations! Pregnancy is all kinds of wonderful and strange and exciting and scary. For the most part, I really loved being pregnant. I'm not saying there weren't moments, because there were definitely moments. But my attitude toward pregnancy was a positive one, and I always looked for the humor in whatever was happening. I think that helped me enjoy my pregnancies, especially when I came across something that caught me off guard, which happened quite a bit.

Sometimes, those off-guard moments happen even before you're pregnant. If you are married, people start asking when you are having a baby even before you've sent thank-you notes for your wedding gifts. And they seem to have no idea that what they are asking is: 1) rude, and 2) none of their business.

When my husband and I first got married, I was peppered with this question repeatedly by a neighbor. We lived in a condominium where the exterior front doors faced one another in a courtyard, and her door was directly across from ours.

This lady was well-intentioned, but we were more acquaintances than friends, so she wasn't exactly someone with whom I would discuss my uterus.

One time she even said in her scratchy voice that made me wonder if she might secretly be the witch from Hansel and Gretel, "Oh, is that a little bump there I see on your belly?" To which I replied, "No, lady, that's a FOOD baby, but thanks for making me feel fat by asking if I am pregnant when I'm not!"

Okay, so I didn't say that, but I wish I had. The truth is I was stunned into silence and just muttered, "Uh, no," and scurried away.

Later, when I actually *was* pregnant, we went to great lengths to hide it from her. When we bought our crib, we had to carry this huge, cumbersome box down the outdoor stairs to our front door. When we got near her door, we laughed and started the power-shuffle to cram it in the door before she could see the big "CRIB" letters on it.

Okay, enough about us. You should know there is a little pre-bump fat phase.

When you are starting to show, people will suspect you are pregnant, but won't want to ask you about it directly. So you will notice folks looking at you and wondering if you are expecting or just eating a few too many snack cakes. I got this question a lot in the cafeteria at work — I guess because I was not hidden away in my cubicle.

The fat phase question goes like this, "*Sooooo... what's new?*"

Then it's up to you if you decide to spill the beans or keep them guessing by reaching for a donut and saying, "Noth'n."

When you are pregnant, you want to tell people when *you* want them to know, not when they ask. Which brings us to...

Telling People

When you find out you are pregnant, you pretty much want to run from the pee stick to the nearest phone, but consider keeping it to yourself (and your spouse) for a day. It's one of the best secrets you will ever know. Plus, it gives you time to evaluate, if you haven't already, whom you want to tell and when you want to tell them.

If you can, I recommend waiting twelve weeks before you tell people — just to make sure everything is okay. Personally, I didn't want to have to share bad news after good if things didn't go well.

Fortunately, everything was fine, but I am still glad I waited to tell the masses.

What?! You mean I can't tell anybody?! Well, I didn't say that. Just don't tell your extended friends and family at first.

I was about to burst with the news so I told a girl at work and then mostly complete strangers or people I didn't know very well, like a cab driver and a girl I sat next to at a banquet. As it turns out, the girl at the banquet was newly pregnant, too. We ended up becoming friends and visited each other in the hospital when we had our babies. We are still friends today.

Mommyhood will connect you to others in ways you never expected.

For our first pregnancy, we made a video to tell my husband's side of the family. It was a recap of something fun that happened at Christmas. And at the end, we had a page that said "Coming Soon — a Bert and Heather Re-Production..." and then the ultra-sound picture.

The next Christmas, my sister and her husband wanted to play us something they had recorded from the radio. But that was just a ruse, as it turned out to be the heartbeat of my nephew-to-be.

I found out about my second pregnancy when my husband was away on a business trip. It was killing me to wait, but I didn't want to tell him over the phone. It was almost his birthday, so I bought some prenatal vitamins and put them in a box. Our daughter and I made cupcakes and gave him the wrapped gift when he got home. So, there are lots of creative ways to tell your significant other or loved ones that you are expecting.

If you are working, you also need to think about when to tell your employer. I told mine at twelve weeks after we let our friends and family know. Your employer needs to know so they can plan for your maternity leave (or departure if you're not coming back). And you will have doctor's appointments to work into your schedule. You'll also want to consult with your boss or human resources department about benefits and paperwork that needs to be completed. If you're planning to breastfeed, ask if there's a lactation room where you can breast pump when you return to work. If there's not, perhaps you can solicit help in getting one set up; all you need is a door you can lock, a comfy chair, and a small fridge (though a sink is also quite handy).

Speaking of telling people at work — you just never know if the folks around you are struggling with pregnancy. For example, I was at work when I felt the first kick and said something to the person next to me in the copy room. He was totally silent and then hinted to me that he and his wife had just lost a baby.

Oy! That's when I realized I had to be careful when talking about my pregnancy. Not that I didn't have every right to be over the moon at the first flutter or anything else pregnancy-related. I was, but after that, I paid more attention to how I handled the good news with people I saw every day at work.

This is true of other people in your life as well. You might find that you and your friends all started to get married around the same time. And then come the babies. But there's usually someone in the bunch that can't conceive when or how she wants.

So, be happy, but be aware of others. People will react to your news in different ways.

And one last thing to note about telling people you are expecting: This kind of news travels quickly. Be aware that the people you tell are probably going to tell other people — even if you tell them not to.

A Word of Advice About Advice

Well, since we have covered how you tell the good news and how folks receive it, let's talk about the dumb things people say when they find out you are pregnant.

Complete strangers will offer you and your spouse unsolicited baby-having, child-rearing advice right along with the change for your cheeseburger. This advice runs the gamut from useless to completely wrong. Not that it is always without merit, but how the little old lady at the grocery store used to do things is not necessarily how things are done today.

One of the most common things people ask you when they learn you are expecting is whether or not you plan to nurse your baby. And in many cases, it doesn't even matter what you say to the person — they are just waiting for their turn to talk so they can give you unsolicited advice or commentary about breastfeeding.

Honestly, it's hard enough to navigate uncharted territory without random idiots giving you their two cents, but that's just how it goes.

And, I should tell you up front that unsolicited advice and being judged by other parents is just a part of being a mom. It happens all the time in everyday life — from how you handle parenting situations to whether or not you nurse to what choices you make for childbirth.

But here's the deal — what you do is your business. **You do not need to discuss, explain or defend your decisions.**

I know when you're expecting there's a lot to wrap your mind around, and you don't know what you're supposed to think about things, and you're excited, so you're going to want to talk about it.

Tips

☆ *Look for common-sense moms to talk with about your pregnancy.*

☆ *If someone has cornered you and is pummeling you with nonsense, just interrupt them to excuse yourself to go to the restroom. You're pregnant so you can get away with that.*

Mum's the Word on the Baby Name

When we were expecting our first child, someone asked me if we had been thinking about any names. I told them a name and they immediately told me they didn't like it (as if I was asking for their opinion — which I was not). So it didn't take long for me to realize the name would just have to be a secret until the baby arrived.

Another thing I learned is that it's not a good idea to name your child one thing and call them something else. It really creates confusion at their doctor appointments and when you fill out documents of any kind. Plus, it is confusing for your child and his or her little friends at school. I did it, but, for what it's worth, I wouldn't do it again.

Going to the Baby Doctor

Choices, Choices

Start by researching various childbirth options. Basically, your choices are between natural vs. medicated and home vs. medical facility delivery. Natural means you don't use any kind of pain-killer during labor or birth; medicated implies incorporating opiates or an epidural for pain.

If your gynecologist isn't an obstetrician (OB) as well, you need to find one. Ask your current gynecologist or a friend (one who will keep your secret) for recommendations. The kind of birth you want will influence the doctor you choose. If you want a natural childbirth, find an OB that is enthusiastic about and supportive of your plan. Some moms opt for a doula in addition to an OB; others opt for a midwife instead of or in addition to an OB. Each choice has different rewards and risks; as with all things in your pregnancy, do what's right for you. All doctors have different personalities (from professional to nurturing, serious to funny) and philosophies; find one that you click with on all levels.

Alright, so let's talk about the role of doulas and midwives. A doula's job is to provide support to a woman both during and after her pregnancy. A midwife is a person trained to deal with low-risk pregnancies and birth; accredited midwifes can manage a natural childbirth at home or in a hospital. So there are lots of options.

We chose a practice with a team of doctors and planned to have a vaginal birth at a hospital with an epidural.

One of the things I didn't realize is how OB practices with multiple doctors work. Basically, you see various physicians for your checkups and then when you go into labor, you get the doctor from that practice that is on call at the time. Actually, it was good for me to have access to different doctors. I asked lots of questions and got lots of information from several different sources. Plus, I wanted to check everyone out, so I was familiar with my delivery doctor on the big day.

You also want to do your homework about how much all of this is going to cost. Our kids were born in different states, each under a different insurance plan. The patient obligations for my son's birth were higher so we paid fees in advance over time. So no two birthing costs are alike — at least they weren't in our case.

Okay, once you settle on a doctor, you schedule your first visit…

The First Appointment: The Wand

At your first appointment you fill out a mountain of forms and then the fun begins. They take blood and urine to confirm your pregnancy, do the initial weigh-in, etc.

This is not typical, but after that we went to the hospital for a viability sonogram. *SWEET! I am going to get to see my baby!* I thought. *It's going to be just like in the movies! They will put some goo on my belly, and show me my kiddo!*

I remember being all dreamy lying there on the table when the technician picked up what looked like a white microphone and put a condom on it right in front of me.

She had my full attention as she squeezed what seemed like an entire tube of lubricant on it and reached for the bottom of my hospital gown…

And *THAT* is how I learned that early sonograms are vaginal.

We saw our little blob of a baby and a tiny fluttering heart, and it was really cool. It was also a big moment for my husband. I think he was still in denial that we were actually having a REAL baby until he saw it with his own eyes.

I think it feels real to us girls sooner because it is our body, but for the guys it just seems like a concept until there is proof. And a sonogram is undeniable proof. Needless to say, that appointment was very memorable.

Once all the initial procedures are taken care of, you schedule your first regular checkup.

First Regular Checkup: Doppler® Heartbeat & Weigh-In

Regular checkups typically occur every four weeks and begin with a weigh-in, followed by peeing in a cup. Then they put you in a room where you wait for the physician while looking wide-eyed at posters and diagrams of the female reproductive system.

The rest of the appointment usually involves listening to the heartbeat followed by a question-and-answer session. And later in your pregnancy, when your belly emerges, the doctor or physi cian's assistant will start to measure your belly top-to-bottom in centimeters at each visit.

At our first regular checkup, the physician's assistant pulled out a little Doppler® machine and asked if we wanted to hear the heartbeat. We were stoked!

She proceeded to put the little wand on my belly and began to move it around. Nothing. She moved it again, and nothing. I watched her like I watch flight attendants on the plane to know if I should be freaking out. She had a pretty good game face as she tried spot after spot looking for a heartbeat.

Silence.

"Is my baby dead!?!?" I whispered because I couldn't bear to say it out loud. My husband was saying some Hail Marys over in the corner when she cheerfully spoke, "Sometimes it's just too early to hear the heartbeat."

I looked at her, mentally grabbed her by the lapels and thought, *"Don't you think it would have been a good idea to mention that UP FRONT. LADY!"* And just as my fear was ratcheting up another notch we finally heard the fast little thump of a heartbeat. Whew! I mean WHEW!

Can you say anxiety? That dreamy first-heartbeat moment just about gave me a heart attack! Thankfully, all was well, but I sure wish I had known it could be hard to find the heartbeat when you are newly pregnant.

Moving on. I should probably warn you that peeing in a cup gets harder the bigger your belly gets, but you will have plenty of time to hone your pee-in-a cup skills as you go along.

But the worst part about the visits is not peeing in a cup; it's the weigh-in. Or it was for me thanks to my ice cream habit.

Toward the end of my pregnancies, I would purposely wear light clothes and take my shoes off before stepping on the scale. I developed quite the complex about my pregnancy weight.

On that note, I would like to speak now to the slim pregnant women (you know who you are). If you eat like a pig but don't gain any extra weight during your pregnancy, don't talk about it to us porky pregos — it's just mean.

About 11-13 Weeks: Genetic Screening

Many women choose a combined test for Down syndrome and other genetic issues; the combined means an ultrasound and blood tests. A friend of mine says that with all three of her pregnancies she opted for genetic tests so she'd have time to prepare and educate herself if the baby had a disability.

We didn't do the screening because we preferred not to know if there was a problem. We just hoped everything would be okay, and, thankfully, it was.

Tip

 The ultrasound tech might even venture a gender guess at this visit if you ask them very, very nicely.

End of First Trimester: Relax a Bit

Your chances of having a miscarriage are much lower in your second trimester, so there's a certain comfort in passing this mark. And if you have problems with nausea it may get better as you head into your second trimester.

Also, at some point you might experience "Prego Brain" where you are mentally dull for no apparent reason. I remember hastily getting on my shoes and grabbing my purse and keys. I walked over to the door with a purpose and then asked myself. *Wait! Where am I going, again?* I had NO idea! So I went and sat on the couch in my coat until I could remember.

Also, I would forget about things that were routine in my life, like what day the garbage truck comes or that I was supposed to send a weekly report to my boss (oops!).

Sorry, I've got no advice for this one, girls, other than to try to laugh about it.

Tip

☆ *Try to stay away from sick people when you are expecting. There aren't that many medicines you can take when you are pregnant, so if you get sick, usually you have to just wait it out (and that's annoying).*

About 20 Weeks: Hot Dog or Hamburger?

You will be scheduled for a sonogram so the baby can be checked out visually and measured. This IS a goo-on-the-belly situation like in the movies. And it's absolutely incredible. And fascinating. And you will want it to last for a really long time because there is assurance in visual confirmation that your baby is doing well. Unfortunately, it's over pretty quickly.

The 20-week sonogram is when you typically find out the sex of your baby if you want to know. Techs like to say they're looking for a tiny hamburger bun (girl) or a hot dog (boy). They also like to say the test isn't 100% accurate, which will make you pause — but not fully prevent you — from buying pink fairy curtains.

We were surprised both times and it was so much fun not to know. It added an extra element of excitement (and wagering).

And all those silly wives' tales about how the speed of the baby's heartbeat or how high or low the baby is carried indicate the gender come into play and make you think, even though they are a load of crap and you know it.

I highly recommend being surprised, but I also know a lot of people who thought I was nuts and had to know what they were having. Whatever works for you is what you should do.

About 25 Weeks: Viva Viability

Though it varies slightly depending on the baby's size, this is the time where your baby can survive outside the uterus, though he or she would initially require intensive care. With each passing week, a premature infant's chances improve greatly. Breathe another sigh of relief.

Tip

 The way you feel physically and emotionally runs the gamut during pregnancy. There are definitely periods when you feel really good. So it's important that you take advantage of those times to get as much of the nursery and other prep work done. I have friends who were put on bed rest for one reason or another towards the end of their pregnancies. If that happens to you, you will be glad you hustled to get things organized.

About 28 Weeks: That Orange Drink

When you are about 28 weeks pregnant, your doctor will schedule you for a gestational diabetes test. For me this didn't take place at my regular doctor's office; I went to a clinic for it. They take blood, give you an incredibly sweet orange soda-like drink and then after about an hour they take blood again to see how your body handles the sugar.

If you do have gestational diabetes, the doctor will put you on a modified diet, and you have to monitor your blood sugar levels. Both of my sisters had gestational diabetes, and say it's kind of annoying to have to manage, but not the end of the world.

Tip

 Take a book or some other entertainment to the diabetes test because it takes a while.

The Home Stretch

At the end of your pregnancy you graduate to weekly doctor's visits and that's when you know you are in the home stretch.

At one of the last few doctor's appointments they do a routine screening called a Group Beta Strep test. It's similar to a pap smear experience, with an extra added bonus — they also swab your rectum. Yes, you read that correctly, but it's quick and not a big deal. I was told most of the time the test is negative, but even if it is positive what they do is give you antibiotics during labor so it doesn't affect the baby.

Tip

★ *If you're prone to yeast infections and test positive for Group Beta Strep, talk to your doctor about what over-the-counter medicine they recommend for yeast infections. Then — and this is the important part — buy it in advance and have it ready when you get home from the hospital. The reason is that antibiotics you'll get during labor may wreak havoc with the good bugs in your system, making you extra vulnerable to yeast infections.*

Wait! There's one other thing I should mention that might happen at the end of your pregnancy. Before you go into labor, you might pass what's referred to as a "mucus plug." Um, what's that? Basically, it's a large vaginal booger (ew!) that protects the cervix while you are pregnant. Passing it usually means labor is not too far away.

Childbirth Classes

Childbirth classes are all different. Ours were not terribly helpful, but I know I learned a few things I didn't already know, so I am glad we went. And there was definitely entertainment value. For example, we had to bring a pillow to one of our classes to use for some breathing exercises. They asked us to get down on the floor for this and during that process one of the pregnant ladies farted audibly. All the mature people acted like it didn't happen.

And then there was us.

We were DYING to laugh. And you know how the more you try not to laugh, the more you really want to? I swear I blew out some earwax trying to keep it together.

Okay, moving on. Childbirth classes also can be reassuring. For example, seeing an epidural tube in person comforted my sister because it was much smaller than she had imagined.

And some classes include a hospital tour, which is a good thing to do. Touring the hospital was very surreal for me, but useful in that I got to see the place where I would have my baby and ask questions about things like having visitors and parking. You can also take a hospital tour on your own; call your maternity ward for an appointment.

We also took an infant CPR class. This was separate from our childbirth class, but we got the information for it from the instructor of our childbirth classes.

The Birth Plan

Toward the end of your pregnancy, you might want to write a birth plan, which is a document that outlines your ideal birth experience. If you choose to write one, you'll go over it with your doctor, and take it to the hospital when you give birth to make sure everyone is on the same page.

One note of advice: Neither your body nor your baby gives a crap about your birth plan. For your own sake, think of it as only a best-case-scenario guideline and be flexible. At the end of the day, the plan is to have a healthy baby, and there are many ways to achieve that. Also, your doctor has lots of patients, so even though you know your birth plan inside and out, he or she may need to be reminded what's in the plan when it's time to have your baby.

And if writing a formal plan is not for you, that's okay. You can always just discuss what you want with your physician.

Tip

☆ *You can find forms online that will guide you through the process of creating a birth plan. Your OB, midwife, doula and friends with babies will also be able to give you good advice and guidance.*

Your Pregnant Body

Fun With Hormones

Your body will change in many ways when you are pregnant. You might have vivid dreams about all kinds of things. I did, and keeping my baby safe was a recurring theme.

You might also find you are a little extra frisky as those hormones have a party in your body.

Hormones can also affect your skin in many ways. For example, I saw an increase in acne with both of my pregnancies. Avoiding sugar probably would have helped, but you know I didn't do that.

There's another change to your skin that is worth mentioning. It's sometimes referred to as the "mask of pregnancy." This is when a pregnant woman experiences brown spots on her skin. These typically go away a couple of months after you have your baby once your hormone levels even out. I have a friend who had brown spots under her arms and on her ears.

I only had a few faint spots on my cheek. I don't remember

being bothered by them, but there were definitely things that did bother me, which brings me to my next point.

Mood swings are a real possibility. So, don't be surprised if you suddenly need to cry or are cranky for no apparent reason. And you should know that just about anything can trigger a mood swing. For example, when I was pregnant with my second child, my husband, daughter and I were at a mall near Atlanta. We were sitting on a bench and I was happily eating a fresh pretzel when a woman who was standing nearby started to talk to me about all the families at the mall.

Honestly, I was paying more attention to my pretzel until I heard her say, "...because I *know* some of these kids don't really belong with these parents."

Um, excuse me? I thought. At that point, I realized the woman was a complete and total whack job. I found myself reaching for my two-year-old daughter's hand and reeling her in protectively.

Once I had a firm grip on her, I started with some polite please-go-away social cues, but the woman started to get defensive and continued to stand there. That pretty much flipped the switch on my hormones. I looked her dead in the face and firmly said, "Listen... you need to move it along, lady."

My husband's eyes bulged and he looked down. I don't know if he was embarrassed or just worried I would turn my wrath on him next.

She looked at me in shock and disbelief but still didn't move. So I stood up, raised my chin slightly and in a go-ahead-make-my-day kind of way I quietly said, *"Move it along, lady."*

So, in summary, you just never know what might trigger a mood swing. Verbal karate at the mall is just one of the ways you might experience the joy of pregnancy hormones.

Construction Zone

Your uterus is a construction zone, so expect to feel some minor aches from all the work going on. If it's severe call your doctor, but I had some cramping and weird little pains with both pregnancies, especially early on when every little twinge freaks you out.

No one tells you how much you worry about how your munchkin is doing in there, but there were times I was absolutely consumed with the fear that something would happen to my baby.

All that worry and construction will wear you out. You will feel groggy and want to sleep a lot, almost like you have a cold. Some people even have a runny nose when they are pregnant. Other side effects include heartburn, dizziness, feeling light-headed or having headaches. This is the perfect time to practice taking good care of yourself; slow down, rest when you need to and listen to your body.

Your joints and ligaments may be noticeably affected. I know a couple of women who had joint pains in their fingers when they were pregnant, and one girl I know experienced carpal tunnel as a side-effect of pregnancy. Not everyone experiences those symptoms, but they are still worth mentioning. The one that pretty much everyone experiences is ligament pain in your hips. This is just something that happens as your body changes to accommodate your growing belly.

You should also know your belly will probably itch as your baby grows. Lotion, which you might receive by the gallon at your baby shower, can help.

Tip

 They make a belly band that you can wear during pregnancy to help relieve pressure on your back from your growing belly.

Chow Time

Your doctor will provide you with a list of foods to avoid when you are pregnant. Your diet is really important, so try to eat as well as you can.

I really overate during my first pregnancy. This was partly to stave off nausea, but mostly because I was stoked to have a license to eat. And I did. I was warned to stay away from the ice cream…

but I didn't. Seventy pounds later, I was pretty sorry about it. But I got a lot of it off eventually. (More on this in the section in Chapter Ten called "Fighting the Battle of the Bulge.")

Pregnancy can also lead to cravings and aversions to food. Everyone's different, so it will be fun to discover what you crave (if anything). With my second pregnancy I had major cravings for ham. In fact, my husband started calling our house Hamalot. This was made worse by a work assignment I did at a HoneyBaked® ham factory. It was like a pilgrimage to the ham mecca! I still think of that assignment fondly.

I don't recall having aversions to any foods, but my friends who did mostly had issues with meat. Additionally, your aversions might be triggered by the smell of certain foods.

Tips

⭐ *Someone recommended eating cereal instead of ice cream because it can help satisfy your craving for something cold and sweet. I, of course, did not heed this advice and paid dearly for it.*

⭐ *Basically, if you "eat for two" you might gain a bunch of extra weight like I did. According to the Mayo Clinic website as of this writing, you only need a few hundred extra calories per day for the baby's nutrition. To put that into perspective, that's like eating an extra half of a sandwich and maybe some yogurt.*

Everything is Swell (Retaining Water)

As your pregnancy progresses, you may become puffy with swelling. In addition to your swollen belly, you will notice at the end of the day your feet might be enlarged. Sometimes my legs would swell right along with my feet — so much so that they wouldn't bend very well. Basically, I had fat knees, kankles and sausage toes. There were a few times I stared at my lower body in disbelief, but a sweet rub of the belly helped me refocus on the pudd'n within.

Tips

⭐ *Propping your feet up can help reduce the swelling. I used to prop mine up on an overturned recycle bin under my desk. That's right, the recycle bin is good for the environment and good for kankles!*

⭐ *Avoiding salty foods (like ham!) can help reduce swelling.*

⭐ *When the swelling is in full force and you feel less than beautiful, consider getting your hair done or painting your nails. One note of caution though, I was told a foot massage could stimulate contractions if you are near the end of your pregnancy. And it's probably not awesome to be breathing in nail salon fumes, but I totally did it. So, if you are jonesing for a pedicure, I completely understand — I mean, it's not like you can reach your toes comfortably — consult your physician if you want to be on the safe side.*

Moving Moments

It's hard to describe how awesome it is to experience the movement of your baby inside you. Remember how I mentioned the sonogram is visual confirmation that the baby is okay? The movement is the physical confirmation that the baby is okay. This usually comes in the wide range of weeks 13-25, and it's totally worth the wait! It's so cool and honestly the part of pregnancy I remember most fondly (despite the occasional kick in the ribs!).

It's also how you first experience behavioral patterns in your child — when he or she is active and what your baby responds to as far as touch, light and maybe even sound.

The movements were special to me because they always prompted me to wonder. *Who are you, kid? Are you a boy or a girl? And what do you look like?* I was desperate to see that little face. The suspense was supreme and heightened by the sensations I got when the baby moved. Feeling the baby move is truly amazing, and all that amazing outweighs the challenges and discomforts that come with being pregnant.

Feeling Big

The bigger your belly gets during your pregnancy, the smaller everyone else appears to you. In fact, I was pretty hostile toward skinny people there at the end. I would be at the mall (you know, eating a cookie) and in my mind talking to everyone who walked by, *And I hate you... and I hate you... and I hate you... and I REALLY hate you, size zero who just said you look fat. Here, want some cookie?*

Not only was I hissing at the skinny people of the world, toward the end of my third trimester, I discovered something else about my pregnant body: Breathing and talking can be difficult when you have a baby affecting your lungs. I learned this while giving a presentation to a room full of executives from my company. I found myself loudly gasping for air between sentences. At one point, I turned to the person next to me and said in front of everyone, "You have to talk now, because I can't breathe."

With help from an awesome colleague, we were able to finish the presentation, but until that happened, I had no idea that pregnancy could be a challenge to public speaking.

Tip

 If you are very pregnant and have to give a speech, include videos or present with a partner who can give you time to catch your breath as you talk.

¿Dónde está el Baño? (Frequent Urination)

You would think that having to pee all the time would happen later in your pregnancy. Not so. It happens pretty early on. By about 10 weeks pregnant I was getting up at night to pee.

Speaking of the bathroom, you should also know that iron deficiencies are common in pregnancy, so your doctor may recommend you take an iron supplement. And additional iron in your system can lead to constipation. If the extra iron in your system bothers you, ask your doctor about stool softeners.

Nocturnal You

Finding a comfortable sleeping position can be a challenge as your pregnancy progresses. Some women use extra pillows to make themselves more comfortable. A friend of mine used a body pillow she named "Stan," which I thought was funny. She loved sleeping with "Stan" so much that eventually her husband was relegated to the guest room so she and "Stan" could have plenty of room to cuddle.

Personally, I didn't like the body pillow. After much trial and error, what worked for me was to sleep on my side with a standard pillow between my knees. Later, when my belly got bigger, I used a really mushy pillow between the side of my belly and the bed. The weight of my belly would pull the rest of my body toward the mattress and I found that having a small pillow there helped.

Cramps are also common. I'm not talking about menstrual cramps, I am talking about killer leg cramps. If you get a strong one, you will be amazed at how fast your large pregnant body is up and out of bed while you make involuntary monkey noises until it passes.

Also, there is a central nerve called the sciatic nerve that starts in the lower back and goes down the back of your legs to your feet. Pregnant women sometimes experience sciatic discomfort. It can feel like a shooting pain, numbness or tingling in the lower back, and sometimes the sensation travels down one leg or the other.

Later in my pregnancy, I would get really hot at night. I remember one time my husband was spooning me when I was hot (and not hot in a good way). I love him so much that I just decided to

let him cuddle with me even though I was roasting. But as my temperature started to rise, I pretty much boiled over and startled him with a semi-whispered yet screechy, *"Get away from me!"*
Ah, good times.

Tip

☆ *Avoid sleeping on your back. When you lie on your back toward the end of your pregnancy, the weight of your uterus creates pressure on the veins that move blood from your legs to your heart. I was told it was better to sleep on your side to help reduce that pressure.*

P-p-p-p-p-pow! (Flatulence)

In case you haven't heard, pregnant ladies are like Whoopie® cushions that don't need to be squeezed.

Sometimes when you are pregnant, you really can't control it. So you just have to hope when and if it happens that you are alone, or with someone who will laugh with you about it. And maybe, just maybe, you can harness your flatulence and use it to your advantage. You see, controlled flatulence is like an angry pregnant woman's secret spider venom, to be used on rude or overly skinny people who truly deserve it.

Case in point. One time I was in the checkout line of the grocery store and the woman behind me was all in my personal space. (She also happened to be one of those people who believe deodorant and breath mints are optional.) "Stinky" insisted on writing her check on the little platform while I was still paying for my groceries. She was so freaking close to me that when she talked my ponytail moved.

Despite my overt social cues, she refused to move, so I let her have it. I knocked her back with an ungodly stench from my pregnant body, and I have never been so proud of a fart!

I'm pretty sure she gagged and staggered backwards.

Or maybe that was just all in my head, but let me tell you, it was a really satisfying fantasy.

So with pregnancy comes magical powers — or rather, powers from the magical fruit. Hopefully no one will cross you. But if they do…

P-p-p-p-p-pow! Let 'em have it!

Vomit

Every pregnancy is different. Some women are pukers (and that just sucks). If that's you, I am genuinely sorry. But, hey, on the bright side, maybe you won't gain a whopping 70 pounds because those potato chips reemerge before they can affix themselves to your arse! And if you vomit and still gain weight, let's just hope those sacrifices are enough to ward off any other pregnancy ills.

Oh, and I have no idea why they call it "morning sickness," because it can be anytime or all the time.

I was a minor puker. I only got sick when I went too long without food, which is how I learned to keep snacks in my purse. But a time or two I found myself hungry and out of snacks.

One time, at the doctor's office, I ate cracker crumbs out of the bottom of my purse. To be clear, we are talking about crumbs that were down there with loose change. My husband was horrified, but I was all, "Shut it, fool. And go find me a drink to go with these crackers!"

Tip

☆ *Keep a bag of crackers or other snacks in your car, desk and purse to help with pregnancy nausea.*

One puketastic moment included me pulling over on the side of the road to barf in a bag of receipts that I was taking to work to shred. The puke on my hair got in my contact lens. And in case you were wondering, bile in your eye is really unpleasant. As for the receipts, I just threw them away, deciding anyone who wanted my identity badly enough to dig through vomit could have it.

But the coupe de grace was the time I took my prenatal vitamin and grabbed a healthy container of raspberry Jell-O® on the way out the door to the airport. I was about three months pregnant and flying from D.C. to Tennessee to see my family. On that flight was the new intern at my husband's office. I had met him for the first time that day when we drove to the airport together.

I'm not a good flier under the best of circumstances, but this trip would turn out to be very memorable. In all my years of flying, it was the most turbulent flight I have ever experienced.

Typically, I use airplane barf bags for scared-of-flying poetry paper. But that day, I held onto it for its intended purpose.

Oh, no. Ohh, oh, no... here it comes, I thought. The flight attendant was announcing there would be no beverage service due to the turbulence as I opened the bag to let 'er fly.

"Are you okay?" said the concerned intern. I wailed in response, "Gimmie some nnnnapkins!"

Despite the turbulence and the fasten-your-seatbelt sign, he got up and asked for napkins only to be reprimanded by the flight attendant for getting out of his seat. He turned and looked at me. I gave him my best *I-will-CUT-you* look and he turned back around and demanded the napkins. I am so thankful he was there, and, you know, he is a friend to this day.

Tips

★ *Don't take a prenatal vitamin on an empty stomach (or with raspberry Jell-O®!)*

★ *If your prenatal vitamin makes you feel sick, ask your doctor if there is another kind you can try, or try taking it at night right before you go to bed.*

On another note, you might also discover that pregnancy gives you a heightened sense of smell. This can be a good thing if you smell something you like or a bad thing if you smell something you don't. But for whatever reason, scents will most likely affect you differently when you are expecting.

Another foe to keeping down food can be your toothbrush. In addition to your nose with magic smelling powers, you might also gain an extra-sensitive gag reflex.

Maternity Clothes

Finding the Basics

I recommend you wear your regular clothes as long as possible.

You can find lots of clothes at places like TJ Maxx® or Marshall's® that will work as maternity wear, and they are a lot more stylish and affordable than some of the official maternity garments. Look for longer shirts, jacket-style sweaters and pants with a low waistline. This works pretty well in the early part of your pregnancy, and these will be the first clothes you turn to after the baby is born.

There also is a fabric tube you can buy that you wear over your non-maternity pants to cover a waistband that won't fasten. It buys you a bit of time in your regular clothes (but not that much).

As your pregnancy progresses, you will need to be in maternity clothes. But maternity clothes are expensive, and you only use them for a short time, so I advise against spending too much money on them. If you can, borrow some from a friend and then buy what you need to supplement that. You might also find some bargains on maternity clothes at consignment stores or sales.

When you do go to a maternity clothing store, they have a pillow you can strap on to simulate a pregnant belly. This is fun; it's neat to imagine how you will look when you are showing.

But I have to tell you the truth about that belly pillow. The belly pillow... is a lie. It's not just your belly that will be bigger. Or, at least that's how it was in my case. For example, I tried on a pair of size medium pants with the belly pillow and they fit with room to grow in the belly. I should buy those, right? Wrong! By the time my belly was ready for the size medium pants, my butt and thighs needed a large.

So buy very few things at a time, and don't pick a lot of items that fit at the moment. It really stinks to buy a bunch of maternity clothes only to discover a few weeks later that none of them fit anymore.

Tips

⭐ *Buy maternity clothes that are slightly larger than your current size.*

⭐ *Don't get rid of maternity clothes you have outgrown; you can wear them after you have your baby and are slimming down.*

⭐ *Maternity tank tops are great. I had a black one and a white one and wore them all the time under various tops and dresses.*

Pants are usually the first maternity item you have to buy. Look for black pants in a comfortable stretchy fabric that can be dressy or casual; you will get a lot of use out of them, especially if you are working. In addition to core pieces like the must-have black pants, get several pairs of knit comfy pants and maybe maternity jeans. Skirts are also great — especially if it's warm.

If you work and have to dress more formally, try a black wrap dress and a black wrap top. I wore those a lot and changed them up with accessories and my non-maternity suit jackets (unbuttoned, of course). If you wear tights, get the maternity version — regular tights will startle you by rolling down your belly when you least expect it.

Casual clothes are pretty easy. Just get a few comfortable things and wear the heck out of them.

Tip

 Don't wear maternity shirts before you actually have a big pregnant belly. You will look like a tool.

Unmentionables

Let's talk panties. When your regular undies just aren't cutting it anymore, it's time to get some maternity underwear. They make all kinds (even thongs). At the end of your pregnancy, the ones that are the most comfortable, in my opinion, are the moderate granny panties. When you get to that point, just get them. It's only temporary.

Tip

 Never look at your own bare, pregnant butt in the mirror. Trust me on this one.

Now let's talk about your ta tas. Or should I say TA TAs! Not only are your boobs sore as your body is gearing up for milk production: They're bigger. You are going to need a bra that fits and is comfortable. Try on some maternity bras to see if you can find one that works for you. You should also look for sleeping bras made for pregnant women to wear at night. There's only a little bit of support, but it's enough to keep the girls in the neighborhood.

Later, you might consider buying a couple of nursing bras if you plan to nurse, but your body will continue to change, so you might wait until you are closer to delivery to select those.

Shoes

Your feet will grow in length and width as your pregnancy progresses. My feet grew a half size in length and stayed that way afterwards. Swelling that made them wider went away eventually.

Though there is not a ton of support in them, it would have been great if I could have worn flip-flops to work, but I needed something dressier. So I found a comfortable pair of sandals and bought them in a few different colors.

Also keep in mind that it is quite difficult to reach your feet in the last few weeks of pregnancy, let alone lace a shoe. Comfortable slip-ons will make your life much easier. A sneaker-like pair for weekends and a nice pair for work are a good investment.

Tip

⭐ *High heels are a bad idea when you are pregnant. Not only is it hard on your feet, legs and back, but also your belly can throw off your balance. One time at work in a dress and heels I fell on my pregnant butt in the hall between two cubicles. Fortunately, I had eaten all that ice cream so I landed on my extra padding and wasn't hurt. But I did roll around on the floor laughing while the guy who saw it happen ran over to help me get up.*

CHAPTER THREE

Gearing Up
for Baby

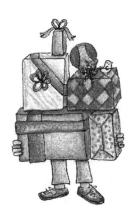

What You Will Actually Use
and What May End Up in a Garage Sale

Going to a baby superstore for the first time when you are pregnant can be very overwhelming. I was intimidated by all the categories and all the options within those categories. The store or web site provides a registry guide to help get you started, but even with that I had no idea what features to look for in baby products.

Tip

☆ *Take an experienced mom with you to the baby store before you register. Ask her to walk through the store with you and tell you what she likes and dislikes about the products she uses. If that mom isn't nearby, take this book with you and go ahead and register. Then ask a friend to look at your registry online to give you some guidance.*

When it comes to registering for baby gear, there's one thing I want you to know: A lot of people have gone to a lot of trouble to convince you that you will be a better mom if you buy X, Y and Z. Well, I'm here to remind you that the human race has survived for centuries without the aid of a diaper wipes warmer.

That said, there are many really useful baby gear items. Here's my take on what gets the most use.

Things You Will Use Right Away

Pack-'n-Play®

Also called a portable crib or a playard, Pack-'n-Plays® are 3' x 4' collapsible pens with high mesh sides and a thin mattress. You want it to have a light, a vibrate feature and music. You also want a bassinet level for when your baby is very small. I never used the Pack-'n-Play® changing-table, but some people do. You may want a Pack-'n-Play® for each level of the house so the baby always has a safe place to play nearby when you need your hands free. These can be purchased used relatively inexpensively.

Swing

Consider the kind that swings from side to side as well as front to back. Not every kid is a swinger, but the right swing can really improve your quality of life if your baby likes to swing.

We put our newborns in the swing but made sure their heads were supported. (Most swings come with a head support, but if you don't have one you can probably get one at a baby super-store.) You will want to use the slowest setting and check the baby often until both of you get the swing of things.

Tips

☆ Consult your swing's instruction manual to make sure you are following all the recommended guidelines.

☆ Swings and other baby devices require batteries – lots of batteries. You will go through more batteries than you ever imagined, so you might as well stock up on a variety of them. Later, you graduate from battery-powered baby gear to battery-powered toys. So you will absolutely use your stockpile (and then some).

The Ultimate Crib Sheet®

In order to get a crib sheet on a crib mattress, you pretty much have to take the mattress out of the crib. And those sheets are so snug, it can be really frustrating under the best of circumstances.

Now, imagine it is 4:00 a.m. and your darling angel has just had the blowout of the ages.

[Ultimate Crib Sheet® enter stage right].

Okay, this is the greatest! You put a regular sheet on your crib mattress. Then you put The Ultimate Crib Sheet® on top of that. It is a flat sheet that has snaps around the edges, which attach to the spindles around your crib. It is soft on top and rubbery on the bottom.

When your baby has a poop explosion during the night, all you have to do is rip off this amazing top sheet and you have a clean bed ready to go. Seriously, this will save you some cursing. I would suggest you register for at least two of these. That way, when one is in the wash you have another to put down. Plus, if your crib converts to a toddler bed — you can continue to use these through potty training.

Bouncy Seat

Bouncy seats are baby-sized chairs with a lap buckle. They sit right on the floor, usually have music, vibration, and overhead toy features, and are quite light. The vibrate feature is particularly handy if your baby is fussy. It can also help them fall asleep. Additionally, we used it when we started to give our baby rice cereal.

Since bouncy seats can be used with very small infants, this is a great way to be hands-free while your new baby is safe and entertained. This is also helpful because it is easily portable. I also used it to bring my baby into the bathroom with me so I could take a shower.

Baby Bathtub

It's a good idea to get one. Talk to your friends about which ones they like. But know that, in general, it's going to work for its intended purpose. These aren't very expensive, so I would probably just get a new one. That said, babies outgrow them after just a few months, so a second-hand shop is likely to have tons of them.

Baby Carriers and Slings

We had the BabyBjörn® and not a sling, but I know people who love their slings, so ask around. I actually didn't use our carrier as much or as long as I thought I would, because babies grow so fast and there is a weight limit. Also, some babies like it and some babies don't, so this might be something you borrow from a friend or look for at consignment. If you choose to buy a knockoff version, take it out of the box and try to put it on before you buy or register for it. If it requires a Ph.D. to get the thing on, you don't want it. I have friends who use the Ergo® carrier and love it. One of the big advantages of it is that it can be used for a newborn (with a special insert) to kids up to 40 pounds; older children can be carried in either the front or in back like a backpack.

Diaper Bag

If your child will go to a babysitter or childcare facility, you will get a lot of use out of a diaper bag. You need it to move bottles and baby supplies back and forth.

When we were out and about as a family, we used a diaper bag for a while with both our babies, but I never liked carrying a diaper bag that looked like a diaper bag. Eventually, we got to the point where we didn't need to have as much baby stuff on hand, so I would pack the bag, keep it in the car and only carry a few essentials in my oversized purse.

I will say that they do make some diaper bags that don't look so bad. Just keep in mind your husband needs to be able to carry it and not look like an idiot, so you might want to avoid the polka dots.

Also, a backpack makes a handy diaper bag when you're going to be doing some walking and need to keep your arms free to manage the baby, like in the airport or at the mall. (See Chapter Eight, "Going Places With a Baby," for what goes inside.)

Receiving Blankets

These are used to swaddle your newborn baby. Wrapping them

up snugly can be calming for newborns. It is my understanding that this is because the cozy feeling reminds them of being in the womb.

Some babies like to be swaddled for a while, but for both of mine it was just two weeks or so. Still, you'll want a few receiving blankets. They are a common gift; you most likely will get them whether you register for them or not. I wish they sold the kind that you use in the hospital, and which the hospital provides. Those were better for swaddling because they were slightly bigger than the ones I got from the store. There also are swaddling blankets you can buy with Velcro® on them to keep your baby wrapped tightly. We never used one, but my sister had one and liked it. Her baby would wake up if he got out of his swaddled blanket, so the Velcro® blanket helped her baby sleep. This is the kind of thing you can pick up later if you need it.

Pacifiers

Surprise! They come in different sizes. (I had no idea.) Start with the newborn size. My husband and I have video of us shoving this enormous pacifier in our daughter's mouth after she rejected it over and over and over again. We just kept shoving it in as we didn't realize the size was wrong for her. It's embarrassing to watch our rookie mistake, but we didn't know! You might get a couple of different styles to see which one your baby likes before buying a whole bunch of one kind; babies have preferences. You also will need a few tethers and pacifier covers.

Tip

☆ *If your newborn baby has a hard time holding onto a pacifier – a nurse once told me to position the pacifier on the roof of my baby's mouth to help them latch onto it. It totally worked.*

Onesies® and SleepSacks®

Onesies® are a one-piece baby outfit that can be long- or short-sleeved that does not cover the baby's legs. Onesies® are a staple baby garment and can be worn alone or underneath other clothes. They make a long-sleeved version that has cuffs that fold over the baby's hands.

If it was cold, we would put our babies in those at night with pants and socks and a hat. We also used something called a Sleep-Sack® wearable blanket, but preferred the jersey fabric to the fleece version because our baby would get too warm.

Tip

☆ *Newborns tend to scratch themselves with those tiny fingernails. In my opinion they don't do this long enough to pay money for a product to prevent it, so this is when the onesies that have the cuffs that fold over their hands are helpful. This also keeps their little hands warm. If you don't have those, put socks on their hands.*

Diapers

I have used the cheaper diapers, and they typically work. However, it is my opinion that when I used them there was more wetness against my baby's skin. The urine odor seemed much stronger to me, too. Note: There are tons of diaper coupons out there. Find them. Use them. You should also explore online discount programs available through sites like Diapers.com and Amazon.com, which offer free shipping for purchases over a certain amount.

Cloth diapers are also an option. They've come a long way from the dishcloth-and-giant-pin version our grandmothers endured; some are even part-disposable.

Fortunately (or, unfortunately), you'll be changing thousands of diapers and if you want to will have plenty of opportunity to experiment with different types.

Tips

⭐ *Don't stock up on newborn-size diapers; you may not need them. We had a big baby and ended up starting with size one.*

⭐ *Get a small basket (with a handle) in which you can keep diaper-changing items. This is a good thing to keep in your living room or places where you spend lots of time. Plus you can take it with you if you move to another room.*

⭐ *When the diaper starts leaking, it may be time to switch to the next size diaper.*

⭐ *While you will want to change your baby's diaper when it's soiled to avoid diaper rash, it's not necessary to wake your baby up in the middle of the night to change a pee diaper unless it is really full. Changing your baby's diaper during the night can wake them up and make it a challenge to get them to go back to sleep. That said, if your baby has pooped, you should totally change the diaper.*

Diaper Cream

When the baby has a diaper rash, zinc-based cream applied at each diaper change is effective. For regular use, baby petroleum jelly works great and is far cheaper than boutique salves.

Pain Reliever/Fever Reducer

Talk to your pediatrician before your due date about what kind they recommend, what dosage they advise for your baby's anticipated weight, and under what circumstances it might be needed. It's better to have a fever reducer on hand if you need it than to have to search for an open pharmacy at 3:00 a.m.

Thermometer

You need a digital ear or temporal artery thermometer (the kind you rub across baby's forehead) for quick checks; both are easy to use when the baby is fussy or asleep. You also need a regular digital thermometer you can use under the arm or rectally if you have to (ugh!), which is still considered the most accurate temperature measurement. They make disposable plastic covers for thermometers.

Burp Cloths

Your baby will spit up, so you will want to have burp cloths or, ideally, cloth diapers on hand for this purpose. They are more absorbent.

Detergent

Baby detergent works well, but it's expensive. Ultimately, I just switched to a detergent free of dyes and scents for all of our laundry. It's easier than trying to wash baby stuff separately. Plus, it's not a bad idea for my whole family to avoid perfumes and dyes in our clothing.

Grooming Kit

You will need a tiny nail file and clippers. Avoid the clippers with newborns and just file the nails. When the baby is a little older, use the clippers. It's easier to cut their nails when they are asleep, by the way. Warning: It's so easy to nip their little skin, and you will feel terrible if you do. But take heart, it happens to the best of us.

Poop Bags

There are scented plastic bags you can buy and keep in your car or diaper bag to use for dirty diapers.

Washcloths

You will use them through toddlerhood. Get plenty (fifteen or so). The little flimsy ones are not very absorbent, so keep that in mind.

Toys

It's going to be a while before your kiddo needs much, but a baby mirror, stacking cups, some toys that clip onto the car seat carrier, and a wrist rattle are all winners for early on.

Activity Mat

This is great for "tummy time," so babies can practice holding up their heads and entertaining themselves. Plus it's portable, so it's also a good way to keep your baby off a floor that might not be the cleanest.

Breast Pump

If you are going to nurse you will most likely want a dual breast pump. I paid an exorbitant sum (around three hundred dollars) for one and was very happy with it. You can also rent one from the hospital. But be advised, even a brand new one can be hard to return, so you might want to make sure nursing will work for you before you get it.

There are two categories of pumps: single-user open-circuit pumps are what you buy from the store; and, closed-circuit pumps are what you rent from a hospital. The manufacturers of the pumps say more than one person should not use a single-user pump; they contend harmful bacteria can make its way to your baby through a single-user open-circuit pump. So, if you plan to use a pre-owned one, just be aware of that concern and read up on it beforehand.

Also, I went online and got a car plug-adaptor for my pump, which I highly recommend.

Bottles

As with pacifiers, your child might have a preference. Get a couple of different kinds first and try them out. Our babies didn't seem to care. We ended up liking the Playtex® Drop-ins® because you can squeeze the bag underneath to get all the air out of the bottle. Plus, using the drop-ins meant less bottle-cleaning for us.

Tips

☆ *Minimizing the amount of air your baby swallows will help reduce gas and tummy aches, so be quick to pull the bottle away when it's empty so they don't swallow air. If taking the bottle away when it is empty is frustrating for baby, but you know they have had enough and will probably spew if you give them any more, be ready with a pacifier after you burp them. Also, some brands of bottles are specifically designed to minimize air bubbles.*

☆ *Bottles come with fast- or slow-flow nipples. When your baby is frustrated because they can't suck the liquid down fast enough, it is time to try a faster-flow nipple. Just be careful when you make the switch: Baby is used to sucking hard for the milk, so the first use of a fast-flow nipple is sort of like shot-gunning a beer.*

☆ *You might see bottles and other plastic baby products that are labeled Bisphenal A (BPA) free. BPA is a chemical shown to have a wide range of negative health affects, particularly if ingested at an early age. BPA is banned for use in baby bottles in the U.S., Canada and Europe.*

Hands-Free Nursing Bra

If you are planning to breastfeed and purchase a pump, consider a hands-free nursing bra. This is a bra that is designed to hold the suction cups from a breast pump so you can be hands-free.

Nursing Pads

If you plan to nurse, you will need nursing pads, which are small, circular pads — similar in concept to a panty liner — that you wear inside your bra to catch any milk that leaks from your breasts. It can take some trial and error to figure out which kind you like best. You just want to make sure you won't be able to see the shape of it on the front of your shirt.

You probably will just need them while your body's milk supply regulates in the first few weeks. And you won't need them at all if you are not planning to nurse. Note: Don't register for these. They are readily available at baby stores, pharmacies and most grocery stores in the baby department.

Lanolin

If you're planning to breastfeed, lanolin is essential. It's a thick yellow goo that keeps your nipples from getting dry and cracked between feedings.

Gel Pads

These are tiny ice packs that you can use to soothe breasts and nipples that are sore from nursing your baby. You wear them in between nursing sessions inside your bra.

Sterilizers

There are lots of gizmos for sterilizing, so this just comes down to personal preference. I used the dishwasher and then sterilized the nipples and pacifiers in a microwave steam bag. It's meant for breast pump parts, but I used it for other things, too. You put the pacifiers and nipples or breast pump parts in this bag with some water and nuke it. Then dump the water and let the parts air dry. It's easy and inexpensive. Note: You still wash the parts first, and then use the steam bag to sterilize them. Also, if you have a really powerful microwave, reduce the power when you use the bag so you don't overheat and warp your breast pump parts.

Dishwasher Basket

There are special baskets that go in your dishwasher that have a lid so you can wash baby stuff without it getting destroyed or lost in the bowels of the dishwasher. If you choose to hand-wash, a bottle drying system for your counter can be helpful.

Nursing Pillow

A Boppie® is that C-shaped pillow that the baby can rest on while you are nursing or bottle feeding. It's also handy when your baby first starts to sit up but is still somewhat unstable. You can sit baby in the middle of it for support, with supervision.

There are a lot of people raving about a nursing pillow called My Brest Friend®. It is a pillow that secures to your belly and is flatter, which is supposed to make breastfeeding positions more comfortable for mom and baby.

Formula

If you are planning to use formula, you may be given a small supply from the hospital to get you started. You may also want to pick up a small container to have at home. Keep the receipt just in case the one you buy is one that doesn't work for your baby.

Tip

 You can also go online in advance and register for free samples and coupons from formula makers.

Car Seats

When the baby grows out of the infant carrier, you will need a car seat. Unfortunately, these can be super-expensive. And if you have two cars, you will need two of them. Even though you don't need these right away, I suggest you go ahead and register for them while people are in the mood to buy you stuff. And I recommend you get the big ones (those that can hold a child up to sixty pounds). They might seem enormous when your baby first uses them, but when your child is bigger and you don't have to spend a boatload to upsize your seats, you will be glad.

If the super-expensive ones are too, well, super-expensive, keep in mind that all child car seats meet very stringent federal safety requirements; it's just that the best seats are much easier to install, have straps less likely to twist, may be more comfortable for the child and may offer additional safety features such as extra side head protection. The safest car seat is the one that fits your car, fits your baby, and is installed correctly.

Tips

☆ *Car seats have expiration dates, so if you are buying a used one, be sure to check the date on it. On our car seats, the date is located on a sticker on the underside of the seat frame. Also, if you are planning to use a second-hand car seat, be sure the seat has never been in a car that's been in a wreck; like bike helmets, their safety structures are compromised by impact.*

☆ *Fire station personnel are trained to ensure your car seats are properly installed in your car. If you aren't sure how to install it, or just want to make sure you have done it correctly, consider a visit to your local fire station. You can also search for a car seat inspection station through the National Highway Transportation Safety Administration at www.nhtsa.gov.*

Infant Carrier/Stroller Combination

An infant carrier is a car seat that snaps out of a base that stays mounted in your car. They are handy because you don't have to unbuckle your sleeping baby when you get out of the car. You just unlatch the carrier, attach it to its stroller or lug it around by its big handle, and go. But choose wisely. This is when you really need to do your homework. After you have determined what you want in terms of safety, you should consider the weight of the infant carrier. You will have to carry that plus your baby. If it is heavy without a baby in it, you might want to keep looking. Also, if you have more than one car, factor in the cost of an extra car seat base.

You will probably have the stroller through toddlerhood, so think about what your needs might be later as well. Are there cup holders for both you and your child? Is there a decent amount of storage underneath? Will the storage bin be dragging on the ground once you put something in it? When you walk behind it, do your feet kick into the storage bin or wheels? Is the handlebar at a comfortable height? Is the stroller easy to unfold? Is it enormous when it is folded up? Will it make you curse when it's time to put it in the car? Is there a visor that will shield your baby from the elements? Does it turn smoothly and go up curbs easily?

Most new car seats can also be used for infants. If you don't want to re-invest in a seat after a few months and don't mind the inconvenience of unbuckling and hauling a sleeping/cranky baby, skipping the infant carrier is an option.

Other Car Products

I highly recommend that you get an L-shaped plastic cover that goes between the baby's car seat and the actual seats of your car. These help protect the upholstery or leather in your car by catching all the dirt, crackers and other food bits your darling angel will add to your vehicle over time. You won't use these right away, but you might as well go ahead and get some covers that attach to the back of the two front seats. These protect your car from dirty little feet that will eventually reach the back of your seat. They come in standard car interior colors, so they blend in to the interior look of your car.

Lastly, if your vehicle does not have tinted windows, consider adding shades to the interior of your car to keep the sun out of baby's eyes. This will pay dividends when your baby is sleeping peacefully as you drive, and you notice the bright sun is shining into the face of your sleeping infant. We used removable plastic shades that cling to the window on the inside. They also make shades that attach with suction cups. If you use those just make sure the shade latches onto something securely, so it doesn't become a flying object in the event of a crash.

And since your baby will be rear-facing for a while, it's helpful to have one of those car mirrors that lets you see your baby's face in the rear view mirror. That way, when your baby starts to cry, you can see if they have spit up or dropped their pacifier.

Tip

☆ *No matter how much you prepare before your baby arrives, you and your spouse will make what feels like millions of trips to the baby store. You will feel like you should buy stock in the store (or stores) you frequent to get baby goods.*

Things You Will Use in a Few Months

You should still register for gear you don't need right away. If you are concerned about storing them, let someone buy the items for you, then take them back and hold onto the store credit until you need them. There is no sense in tripping over baby gear until you are actually ready to use it. Plus, by the time you need it, the manufacturers may have made improvements.

Booster Chair With Tray

Instead of a traditional highchair, I found an adjustable booster chair with a tray that attaches to the chair to be very convenient. They take up less space and serve the same function. They also are portable and useful through toddlerhood.

Stationary Activity Center

This includes the ExerSaucer® and other big round plastic things in which the baby is supported in a standing position in the middle, a perch from where they can (depending on the activity center) bounce, spin, play and explore a variety of attached toys. Once your baby can hold his or her head up well, this is another great place to put them so you can take a shower, cook and so forth.

Tips

⭐ *If your baby has reached the recommended age for your stationary activity center but is still a little wobbly in there, stuff a sweatshirt in behind them to prop them up.*

⭐ *Speaking of propping up, if your little one is able to sit up, but too small for a restaurant highchair, try putting your purse behind your baby to push them towards the table and strap them in with the safety belt.*

Jumping Station

This is similar in concept to an activity center, but the center of it is supported by bungee cords so your baby can jump to their heart's delight. Starting around five months, your baby will love jumping, so a jumping station is worth having if you have room.

Things That May End Up in a Garage Sale (Or, Things You Can Really Do Without)

Highchair

Highchairs are great because they provide another place to put your baby so you can be hands-free. But mine always seemed to be in the way, so if you are tight on space, consider a booster seat with a tray that straps onto a chair instead.

Diaper Wipes Warmer

While it's a nice idea, in my opinion this is just not practical because you end up changing diapers all over the place and a diaper wipes warmer is confined to one location. If your wipe is cool, you can always warm it up in your hand before you use it.

Infant Carrier Stroller Frame

I don't recommend the kind of infant carrier stroller that's just an empty frame; when your baby outgrows the infant car seat carrier (which will be faster than you can imagine), you will be left with a useless stroller frame. Someone recommended this to me, so I got one. I think I used it once. It just makes more sense to get an infant carrier/stroller combination.

Infant Car Seat Cover

They make warm covers that are made to fit snugly over your infant carrier. Unless you live in a cooler climate and plan to spend a lot of time outdoors with your baby, a blanket works just fine. However, if you live in a place with very cold winters, this is a great thing to have. They even make larger ones that fit on strollers that will keep your toddler warm.

Poop Holder

It is my personal opinion that you can do without the latest, greatest poop holder. Why on earth would you want to store thirty-five or so bowel movements in the room where your precious baby sleeps? You can just put them in your trash and take the trash out regularly.

Tip

☆ *If you get a poop holder, consider one that opens with a foot pedal. And when it's time to empty it, I highly recommend that you take it outside first. Fair warning: it is a stench like no other!*

Changing Table

I am sure there are people who have used their changing tables to change diapers, but I just ended up using the drawers in mine for storage. You will change diapers on the floor, the bed, the couch, the table and even the counter. You can even get a changing pad and use it on a dresser in the room if the dresser is a good height for it. I wished I had just gotten a regular dresser instead of a changing table. I had to go buy one later. Live and learn.

Layette

What is a layette? A collection of baby clothes. And I know it's hard to imagine, but your baby will grow really fast. On one hand, of course you need baby clothes, but on the other hand, keep the following in mind: You can have the cutest collection of three-month-old dresses or suits or cowboy outfits and it's possible your baby will not wear them once, either because the baby will grow too fast or you will be so tired that anything with more than two buttons is deal-breakingly inconvenient. So make sure you have plenty of comfortable, one-piece, season-appropriate clothes that you won't mind throwing away if they get ruined.

Tips

☆ *Look for outfits that zip up. Fastening, unfastening and re-fastening 15 snaps 15 times a day will make you appreciate and seek out baby clothes with a zipper!*

☆ *When you zip your baby's outfit, be sure to do so with your finger between the zipper and your baby's skin to protect them.*

Baby Powder

The experts advise against using talc-based baby powder, because it can be harmful if babies inhale it.

Tip

☆ *Consider faux registry items. A lot of people will want to get you a gift in the range of $25-$50. So, you might consider looking for additional items to register for in this price range (even if you don't want or need them). You can then take those things back and pool your money toward the bigger items you didn't get. If people feel like there aren't a lot of reasonably priced items left on your registry, then they go off and do their own thing. This typically does not work in your favor, as you might get things you don't need and have trouble finding out where to return them.*

Saving Money on Baby Gear

If you have friends who already have babies, see if you can borrow some of the things their child has outgrown.

If you are a first-time mom, the thought of something used might not be your favorite idea. But if it can be sterilized, it's really no big deal. And if you're on a budget, this can save you a ton of money.

Additionally, second-hand baby stores often have the exact same item that boutiques carry for a fraction of the price. Ask an experienced mom where she does her shopping. Just remember to do your due diligence: Research recalls and use your own best judgment before purchasing any used item.

What Goes Into a Rock'n Nursery

When it comes to the nursery, the first thing you should know is that the baby doesn't care. From functionality to aesthetics, the nursery is pretty much for Mom, and only a little for Dad and the baby. After all, Mom is the one nesting and the baby is oblivious to its surroundings for quite a while. So this one's for you, Mom. Make it a special place for you to be with your baby.

Basics You Will Need (in Random Order)

Crib

Be sure to research recalls and read online reviews before you purchase a crib, especially if you plan to use one that is not new. If you purchase a used crib, be aware that federal safety regulations make it illegal to buy, sell or donate drop-side cribs due to suffocation hazard if the drop-side malfunctions. If you are given a drop-side crib, call the manufacturer to see if you can get a kit that will bring the crib up to code.

Consider a crib that converts to a toddler bed. I didn't get a convertible crib because I thought the ones that were available at the time were all ugly. And I generally don't like the look they produce as a full-size/queen headboard, but it would have been nice to have a crib that became a toddler bed.

However, if my husband and I had purchased a convertible crib, when baby #2 came along, we would have had to move our toddler to a traditional bed anyway so we could put the new baby in the crib. So it worked out well to get a basic crib and move our toddler to a traditional bed with bed rails when the time came.

Chair

I did not get a rocker or a glider. I got an upholstered rocker-swivel chair for the nursery and it was a good decision. We used to use it for feedings; now, we use it for story time. Personally, I am glad I got a comfortable piece of furniture rather than a wooden rocking chair or nursery glider. It has definitely evolved with us! The only thing I would do differently is to use a lighter color upholstery fabric. Our chair is red. I thought that would hide dirt. The reality is milk, formula and baby vomit are white.

Bookshelf

Depending on your nursery, you are going to need some storage for baby stuff. Also, it won't be long before you accumulate a number of books, so this is an item that will grow with your child.

Room-Darkening Shades

Since babies sleep during the day, it's helpful to have a way to make the room in which they will sleep dark. I recommend room-darkening roller shades. These are very affordable and can be cut to size at your local hardware store while you wait. I used them under drapes or other window treatments that matched my nursery décor.

Monitor

If you can spring for it, the video monitors are really great. They are useful because you can keep an eye on your baby without going into the room. You don't want to accidentally wake them up! Plus, your baby will continue to take naps for a couple of years, so you will get a lot of use out of an item like this.

Tips

⭐ *If you plan to get a video monitor, you should know that the inexpensive ones can produce a lot of static, and a loud baby monitor is not ideal. Check product reviews to make sure you get a quiet one.*

⭐ *Also, look into a digital one with encryption so other people can't hear what you say on their baby monitors.*

And if a video monitor is not in the budget, a traditional monitor will totally get the job done, too.

Clock

If you are nursing or want to know if it's time to make a bottle, you will need to know the time.

Cool Mist Humidifier

Humidifiers are useful when your baby has a cold or if you live in a dry environment. I suggest you get a decent one. You don't have to break the bank, but don't get the cheapest one on the market; a cheap one can make your floor wet. And make sure the one you buy has replacement filters that are readily available. I had to buy a whole new humidifier once because I couldn't find a replacement filter for my existing one.

Toy Storage

Get a basket or something you can use to store toys. It will be almost three months before your child can even hold anything, but you won't believe how little time it takes for your child to accumulate toys.

Dimmer Switch

One of the brighter things we did was install a dimmer switch on the light in the baby's room. It is great for late-night feedings and diaper changes. But a small lamp will do as well.

Things You Will Use: A Registry Guide

What You'll Use Right Away:

☐ Pack-'n-Play®

☐ Swing

☐ The Ultimate Crib Sheet®

☐ Bouncy Seat

☐ Baby Bathtub

☐ Baby Carriers and Slings

☐ Diaper Bag

☐ Receiving Blankets

☐ Onesies® and Sleep Sacks®

☐ Diapers

☐ Diaper Cream

☐ Pain Reliever/Fever Reducer

☐ Thermometers

☐ Burp Cloths

☐ Pacifiers

☐ Grooming Kit

☐ Poop Bags

☐ Washcloths

☐ Toys

☐ Activity Mat

NURSING ITEMS

☐ Breast Pump

☐ Lanolin

☐ Bottles

☐ Sterilizers

☐ Dishwasher Basket

☐ Nursing Pillow

☐ Formula

CAR ITEMS

☐ Infant Carrier/ Stroller Combination

☐ Car Seats

☐ Window Shades

☐ Rear-facing mirror

What You'll Use in a Few Months:

☐ Booster Chair with Tray

☐ Stationary Activity Center

☐ Jumping station

What Goes Into a Rock'n Nursery:

☐ Crib

☐ Chair

☐ Bookshelf

☐ Room-Darkening Shades

☐ Monitor

☐ Clock

☐ Cool Mist Humidifier

☐ Toy Storage

☐ Small Lamp

Hurry Up and Wait

As more and more of your pre-baby chores get done, you'll have time to think and wait and dream about your sweet baby.

Toward the end of your pregnancy, you start having weekly doctor visits. When you get to that point, it's almost like someone has just wound the clock and you are now a ticking time bomb.

As I mentioned earlier, weekly visits are the home stretch. Unless you are having a scheduled delivery, at some point your doctor may say something unintentionally cruel to you like, "Pack your bag, it's any day now!"

If you are unbelievably ready to get the baby out of your body "any day now" might make you breathe fire as day after day passes with no baby arriving on the scene.

Or, you're standing there and your belly is so big it's over the state line and some well-meaning idiot co-worker feels compelled to state the obvious. "No baby yet?" You have to choke out a polite laugh while you are thinking, No, Butt-wad! And please, make sure to say that when you see me again tomorrow and I'm *still* pregnant! This is precisely the kind of special moment that led me to fantasize about owning a TASER® electronic control device. (Bzzzzt!)

So, now it's time to hurry up and wait.

Since you have a little more time, you might as well be productive. There's always something else you can do to prepare for the arrival of your baby.

Make-Ahead Meals (Because You'll Be Tired, and You'll Be Hungry)

When you have a baby, people typically bring you food through the first few weeks. It's great, but it only lasts so long. Eventually, your helpers depart and you are expected to juggle this tiny creature that is dependent on you and start doing things you used to do – like cook.

To make things a little easier on yourself, consider preparing a few make-ahead meals to put in the freezer. After all, you are going to go through the ringer of sleep deprivation and you probably won't feel like putting a whole lot of effort into a meal. And meals you make yourself are preferable to store-bought frozen options because: 1) they are much cheaper, and 2) you'll appreciate your regular favorite food when you need a sense of normalcy. It's a good way to nurture yourself in advance.

What to Pack in Your Hospital Bag

☐ Infant Carrier or Car Seat
You (and baby!) can't leave the hospital without it. And whatever you do, make time to install the base well before your due date.

☐ Take-Home Outfit for the Baby
Make sure it's a newborn-size garment. I took a 0-3 month outfit and it was huge. Additionally, you might pack an extra take-home outfit just in case your little bundle has a poop explosion as you are snapping pictures and preparing to leave the hospital. Also, don't forget a hat, socks and blanket.

☐ Your Birth Plan (If you have one)

Tip

☆ *Depending on how much there is to know, you might consider writing up a list of details for family members who will come visit when you have your baby. For example, we included directions to the hospital and parking information as well as the location of the best entrance to get to the maternity ward, security information, etc.*

☐ Pad of Paper and a Pen

Very useful for making lists of people to call or for taking messages or keeping track of gifts and flowers.

☐ Bras

Take nursing bras and disposable nursing pads if you are planning to nurse. If you are not planning to nurse, you will need to bind your breasts (doesn't that sound nice?). So take a sports bra or one of your smaller ones for this purpose.

☐ Pillows

Take one or two of your own pillows. Hospital pillows are like a wad of cheap tissue in a wheat sack. Some literally fold in half like a piece of paper. Put your personal pillows in colored pillowcases so they are easily identifiable as yours.

☐ Something to Wear Other Than a Hospital Gown

Once you have your initial round of visitors (and you get some much-needed sleep) you will want to put yourself together as much as you can. You'll take a shower, put on a little makeup, etc. I was glad I had some stretchy black pants and a top as well as a cardigan long enough to hide my postpartum rump.

☐ Robe and Slippers

You might be roaming the maternity ward while in labor.

Tip

☆ *You might also want to consider getting a pedicure in advance as visitors may be seeing your bare feet in the hospital bed and you don't want to have fugly toes.*

☐ **An Outfit for You to Wear Home From the Hospital**
Second-trimester maternity pants or sweats and a very comfy shirt will get you home just fine.

☐ **Toiletries/Makeup**
People will be taking lots of pictures, and you will be swollen with matted hair. I don't wear much make up normally, but a little lip-gloss and a comb helped me feel better about myself in the hospital.

☐ **A Roll of Soft Toilet Paper**
Some hospital toilet paper is better suited for filing your nails or sanding your deck. So, unless you plan to whittle your recently busted vagina, you might want to grab a roll just in case.

☐ **Maternity Underwear**
Your granny panties' swan song. Hopefully you can graduate to normal underwear again soon.

☐ **Thick Menstrual Pads**
(Clearly, tampons are not an option here.) The pads I was provided were like diapers. You need those at first, but later it's nice to have a less bulky option. The hospital will provide pads, but I was there for a few days. So I was happy to graduate from the thick menstrual pads to some smaller ones I brought from home.

☐ **Video or other Camera and Batteries/Charger**

☐ **Phone and Phone Charger**

☐ **Music/Speakers**

☐ **Glasses/Contacts**

Things I Took That I Didn't Need to Take

⊘ **Snacks for Visitors**

What was I thinking — that I would be hosting a party or something? Hindsight is 20/20. People can get their own stink'n snacks. You might, however, want some for you and your spouse, especially if you have a C-section and are in the hospital for a couple of days. Some maternity wards provide excellent complimentary snacks; asking beforehand could save you the effort of bringing anything at all.

⊘ **Jewelry**

Leave your jewelry at home. One less thing to keep track of.

CHAPTER FOUR

Assembling Your Babycare Team

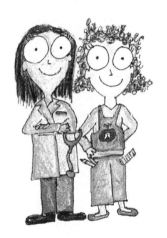

P eople say "it takes a village to raise a child." I would agree. A lot of people will help see to the well-being of your baby. You are going to need a good pediatrician and assistance when you get home from the hospital. And whether you need childcare immediately or not, it's a good idea to understand your options.

For me, the hardest part was trying to figure out what to look for. I had only a vague idea of the questions I should be asking. It sure would have been nice if someone had pointed me in the right direction. So, here are some things to consider as you assemble your babycare team.

Finding a Good Pediatrician

You'll need to find a pediatrician before your baby is born. Get a list from your healthcare provider online and talk to other moms in your area. I recommend you go meet with anyone you are considering. Here are some things to consider as you evaluate pediatricians.

- Ask him/her about himself/herself and the practice. Find out where they went to school and how long they have been practicing. Does he or she have children? It's not a must, but a pediatrician who is also a parent is a plus in my opinion.

- How many doctors are in the practice? At our practice, we see our regular doctor for well visits and if she is not working and we need a sick visit, we will be seen by another doctor in the practice or a physician's assistant. A practice with multiple doctors can be a good thing: Typically, the more doctors, the faster they can get you in to see someone.

- Think about whether you want a male or a female doctor.

- How were you treated by the staff when you called and arrived for your appointment?
- Is the office clean?
- Are there separate sick and well entrances/waiting rooms?
- Is it well-run? You can have a great doctor, but if the office is run poorly and it takes forever to do even a quick visit, that's certainly something to consider. How would you know from an initial visit? One sign is if the waiting room is packed with annoyed parents and kids climbing the walls.
- What kinds of hours do they have? Do they have any weekend hours?
- Is there an after-hours nurse line? What other resources are available through the practice?
- What kind of vibe do you get from the doctor? Will he/she welcome your endless new mommy questions? There are a lot of great doctors out there. That said, beware the condescending pediatrician. That's the last thing you need while you are learning to parent your child (and are hormonal and sleep-deprived).

Once you have selected a pediatrician, you can discuss things like shots, feedings and circumcision.

Okay, pediatrician... check! Now, let's move on to childcare.

What to Look for When Evaluating Childcare Options

Your baby isn't even born yet, and already you have to think about turning them over to someone else! But, unless you are planning to stay home, you have to do it. So start thinking about what's going to work best for you. It can take a while to find the right place, and that place may come with a wait list.

Basically, your two options are in-home care or child development centers. Here are a few generalized pros and cons of each to get you started.

Kinds of In-Home Care:

Babysitter
Your baby is watched by an adult/adults at your home or the home of a caregiver.

Nanny
A nanny is someone you hire as a dedicated childcare provider for your child/children. In some cases the nanny resides in your home.

Nanny Share
A nanny share is when more than one family jointly hires a nanny to care for their children at a location that is designated or rotated.

Child Care Co-Op
A co-op is when parents share childcare duties. Typically, the childcare duties are divided equally and no money is exchanged.

Questions to Ask of an In-Home Childcare Provider:

- How long have you provided childcare in your home?
- Are you a licensed childcare provider?
- Do you know CPR and first-aid?
- Have you ever been arrested?
- Do you or anyone who resides in the home have a history of mental illness? Are you or is anyone who might be in the home with my child on any kind of medication? (Okay, that might seem like an embarrassing thing to ask, but you need to know.)
- Do you or does anyone in your home smoke?
- Where will my child eat, sleep and play?

⊙ Do you provide a curriculum for the children? (You'll want to know that for later).

⊙ Will my child be experiencing any TV or video time, and, if so, how much?

⊙ What other people will be in the house with my baby?

⊙ How many other children do you care for, and what are their ages?

⊙ How much help do you have to assist with the children?

⊙ What happens when you get sick or take a vacation?

⊙ Will you be caring for your own children as well as mine?

⊙ Will my child have outdoor playtime? How often, and for how long? Evaluate the condition of the outdoor equipment and the security of the location.

⊙ Are there pets? (Is there an animal present that could give my child a scratch or a bite?)

⊙ Evaluate the cleanliness and location of the bathroom and diaper changing area. Is the bathroom nearby, so the children won't be out of earshot when the caretaker is using it, or will the caretaker be able to keep a close eye on young children during potty training? How often are diapers changed?

Types of Child Development Centers:

Daycare/Preschool

Daytime care is provided to classes of infant and preschool-age children at a church, school or business location.

Mother's Day Out

Many churches provide childcare programs referred to as Mother's Day Out or Parent's Day Out. In most cases, this is a part-time, paid childcare option.

Questions to Ask at a Child Development Center:

- Is the childcare facility licensed with the state?
- Do you conduct background checks on all of your workers?
- What kind of curriculum do you offer? (You'll want to know that for later.)
- What is the teacher/child ratio?
- How long have the teachers in the infant room worked at this location? What kind of staff turnover do you have?
- What time is drop off and pick up? What if you're late?
- How do you handle conflict between children?
- How do you handle potty training?
- Is there a wait list? (Sometimes a wait list can be a good indicator about the childcare provider.)
- Ask about their security system.
- Do you have a camera system that allows you to view your child online during the day? (This wasn't a deal-breaker for me, but it is a bonus if they have it.)

What kind of childcare should you choose? There is no wrong answer. It's whatever is best for you and your baby.

Sometimes you have to pursue several options and see which one works out. And, unfortunately, what you want is not always available when you want it. So consider creating a top-three list of options. Sometimes you have to go with a top-two or top-three choice while you wait for space availability at your first-choice location.

Not sure where to start? Talk to other moms in your area. Ask about their childcare solutions and what they like and dislike about their situation. Go online and start researching.

Should you look for a place that is closer to home or closer to work? What if your spouse works at the other end of town or commutes somewhere? If so, perhaps closer to home is a better option. Think about who will drop off and who will pick up. It's better if you and your spouse can share this duty, so begin to explore options in those locations.

Once you have your choices narrowed down, make appointments and go tour the facilities. When I was checking a place out, I spoke with parents in the hall or parking lot (in other words, someone who was not a designated reference). Pay attention to safety. Can you just walk right in, or does the security system keep you out? Also, look for cleanliness.

Don't forget to pay attention to the vibes you get from the people in the places you check out. Do the kids look happy? Do the workers look happy? Places with long-term employees can be a good sign that the place is well run.

If you are checking out childcare centers on your lunch hour, keep in mind that naptime is not a great time to tour a facility. If you are leaning toward a place and only saw it during naptime, arrange another visit for when things are in full swing to make sure you have the whole picture.

Also, don't just take the potential caregiver's answers at face value. Check their references. Search online for informal complaints against the individual or location. If the provider is licensed, research any formal complaints filed. Additionally, do a search for registered sex offenders near the facility.

Selecting childcare can be stressful. It is a huge decision. But, once you have done your research and made your choice, there is one less unknown to handle. Hopefully, making this selection (if you need to) will reduce your anxiety as the pieces start falling into place.

Tip

☆ *Go online and do a search for registered sex offenders near your home and childcare location.*

Childcare Quick Comparison

In-Home Care	
Pros	**Cons**
◉ Personalized attention	◉ Less structure/curriculum
◉ Consistency — the caregiver is ultra familiar with your baby's needs	◉ Will this person leave the premises for a chore and take your baby along?
◉ Fewer other kids to make your baby sick	◉ What if the caregiver falls and hits her head?
◉ Home environment	
◉ More schedule flexibility	◉ What if the caregiver is sick or needs a vacation?
◉ Typically more affordable	

Child Development Center	
Pros	**Cons**
◉ Evaluated on a consistent basis by a third party	◉ Increased exposure to illness, although some might argue the child is building up their immune system.
◉ Transparency: other adults see the facility	
◉ Stated policies and procedures	◉ Less attention from caregiver
◉ Your child will be with other kids the same age, and have an age-tailored curriculum	◉ Less flexibility with schedule
	◉ More expensive
	◉ Fees for late pickup
◉ Some childcare centers have great security systems	◉ May learn aggressive behavior
◉ More curriculum-based learning	◉ May pick up bad habits from other children

The Helpers Will Cometh

When you have a baby, it is common for your mom, mother-in-law or a friend to come and help you those first few weeks. While it's really great to have help, it is important for your helpers to know up front what you expect from them.

For me, I wanted my mom and mother-in-law to help take care of things at home so I could figure out how to manage my baby. I was worried everyone would be all over the baby and I would be schlepping around doing the housework. So we had a little talk up front, and when I came home from the hospital with my baby, all was well. I figured out how to care for my baby – I even had experienced moms right in my house to ask timely questions of! – and my mother, mother-in-law and friend eliminated dust bunnies most of the time. Having a conversation like this might not be necessary for you, but it is something to think about.

Single Moms

If you are an expectant mom going it alone, you can totally do this. But you are going to need some help. Find supportive friends and family members that can be with you at the hospital for the birth and stay with you once you get home.

Tip

⭐ *If you need it, the USDA's nutrition program called Women, Infants and Children (WIC) provides formula for moms and food for breast-feeding moms who need financial assistance. I have a friend who had her first child while she was in college and support from WIC helped her get through it.*

I also have a friend whose husband is in the military and was deployed when she had her baby. And I know she received fantastic support from other military wives in addition to the support she received from her friends and family.

CHAPTER FIVE

Childbirth

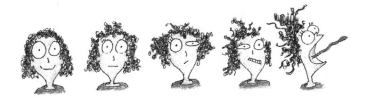

Excuse Me, Please, But There's a Stork Circling Above Your Head

During my prenatal class, the instructor said one in four women have a C-section. I smugly sat there and wondered which of those other women would be having C-sections. Like all first-time moms I had this vision of going into labor and my husband rushing me to the hospital like in the movies. Well, I was one in four who had a C-section.

We found out two days before our baby was due that she was breech —frank breech — which meant she was head up and feet up. I was devastated that my movie-like birthing was not to be. Plus, I had spent a good deal of time worrying about how that baby was going to come out, and now all of that was in vain!

Not only did we learn she was breech, but she was going to be a large baby. The ultrasound technician who confirmed she was breech estimated her at 10 pounds 15 ounces. As those numbers were rattling around my brain, I began to perspire, tear up and get mad at my husband for doing this to me — who wouldn't? (I'm about 5'4," and yes, I had eaten my share of ice cream and chocolate pie during the pregnancy, but surely I didn't deserve this!)

Suddenly the stork with the dainty bundle circling above my head had morphed into pterodactyl struggling to fly a lump the size of a Thanksgiving turkey!

A Word About That Birth Plan

As I mentioned, it's a good idea to have a birth plan. However, births don't always go as planned, so you'll want to mentally prepare yourself to be flexible.

My super-awesome mother-in-law often asks, "Will it matter a year from now?" That is an excellent question to ask yourself when it's time to have your baby and things aren't happening according to the plan.

The goal is a healthy baby and a healthy mom, and the best outcome will result when you can be confident in what you want yet smart and flexible.

Gimme a C... Section!

Fortunately, I only had about eight hours to freak out about the C-section. But as I thought about my enormous baby-to-be, I realized how thankful I should be that my toddler-size baby would be surgically removed.

I didn't have anyone near me who had experienced a C-section, so I was really on my own.

Even if you are planning on a vaginal birth, things happen and you might end up having a C-section. So, here are some things to know about the planned C-section process.

You can't eat after midnight. (This was especially hard for me, as I am a lost member of The Golden Girls™. There is nothing like cheesecake in the middle of the night.)

Your husband will look adorable in scrubs while you look like a light blue pup tent.

Amazingly, you will find yourself reassuring your nervous husband that everything will be okay. This actually keeps you busy and distracted. Plus, you get to reassure yourself in the process.

They hook you up to monitors, and you get an IV, an epidural and a spinal block. During the epidural, you have to hunch forward and be still — as if it is easy when you are a million months pregnant. It feels like cold water being poured into your spine. I guess that took place before the spinal block, because I don't remember what that felt like. A spinal block is a single (numbing) shot, whereas an epidural involves a catheter in your back through which medicine can be delivered constantly.

One thing that did happen before the numbing took effect; a really unhappy nurse at the end of her shift roughly dry-shaved me, um, "down there." I couldn't see it, but my husband later told me it bled. Word to the wise, ladies, ask your doctor if this is something you should consider taking care of beforehand. Not that this is easy either when you are very pregnant. Naturally, as this woman was going to be involved in bringing my baby into the world, I decided I better be super polite. "Yes, dry-shave me some more. I like it. Just don't hurt my baby!"

You'd think I would have remembered evil Nurse Hatchet and taken care of business for my second baby, but thanks to my "prego" brain, I forgot. Fortunately, all was well. My second delivery happened at a different hospital and they used an electric razor, which was no big deal.

They pump you full of fluids through an IV. THAT is why when you see pictures of moms with newborns they look bloated and not quite like themselves. (This is true for a vaginal birth as well.)

The epidural makes your teeth chatter (or, it did mine anyway). Your teeth will chatter as you are wheeled down a hallway in a very surreal experience while you look at the ceiling and begin to feel numb from the chest down.

I remember a nurse saying she was going to go get my dad. I remember thinking "but my dad is in Tennessee!" I only realized after she left that she had meant my husband. That was the first time someone with authority (a medical person) called my husband a dad, and my first real indication that Mommyhood was, in fact, upon me.

Generally the anesthesiologist will start the epidural and anesthesia and then a nurse anesthetist will take over. Our anesthesiologist actually stayed with us the whole time. He and my husband sat on stools near my head. Interestingly, my anesthesiologist looked like Bill Clinton, and my baby was born in the Washington, D.C. area.

My husband was not interested in getting a look at my beautiful spleen. So during the procedure, he and I nervously chatted up our Bill Clinton look-alike to pass the time. And I told the following joke to my doctors during the surgery: "What did the Mama bullet say to the Daddy bullet? ... 'I'm having a BB!' "

They secure your arms. (Not that you can feel to move them anyway. Perhaps that is so they don't fall off the table).

The whole surgery takes about fifteen minutes. I asked my husband when they were going to start and he laughed and told me they were almost done. At this point my body was rocking from side to side as they were getting our baby out. The drugs made me a little clueless.

Moment of irony — the doctor who did my first C-section was new to the practice. So, I spent nine months dutifully meeting all the doctors in the practice just in case they were the one on duty for my vaginal delivery, only to have a complete stranger deliver my baby via C-section. She did a great job, though, so I won't complain.

Incidentally, that technician was really off in her weight prediction. My daughter was only nine pounds, but in the nursery next to all the other newborns she was still quite the hoss.

My second child was also delivered via C-section. During that procedure, I started thinking too much about the numbness. I couldn't feel myself breathing and began to freak out. They gave me some happy juice through the IV, and I calmed down.

Typically, the C-section incision is horizontal and at the top of your pubic hairline. Afterwards, they use tape, staples, glue or stitches on the incision, and then put tape on top of that. After both of my C-sections, all of this was removed before I left the hospital. Warning! The tape hurts like hell when it comes off. If you have staples you don't really feel anything when they remove them because you lose feeling (forever, I think) at the incision.

I was really surprised how fast the exterior incision healed. The inside part takes a bit, and you will walk hunched over like a little old man at first from the pain. Word to the wise — stay ahead of the pain by using the drugs as prescribed. When you are on the meds and not feeling any discomfort, you start to think that you could probably handle a little pain. Don't be a hero! Take your meds if you need them. That said, I only took the heavy meds at first. As soon as I could, I switched to Aleve®. If you are planning to breastfeed, let your doctor know so they can prescribe painkillers that don't affect breast milk.

Warning! Do not underestimate the importance of stool softeners. Many pain medicines are constipating, so stool softeners are absolutely essential. (More information on the importance of stool softeners later in this chapter.)

Post C-section you will also want to avoid stairs. Climbing stairs can pull on the incision area and make you whimper and wince in pain. So, take it slow and you will be feeling better soon.

Also, you should know that after you have a baby, the nurses measure the amount of urine you produce to ensure your bladder is functioning properly. They do this by hooking a plastic measuring cup to the toilet that catches your urine.

Lastly, frank breech babies delivered via C-section may have perfectly round heads, but be aware they sometimes have hip problems. Because their hips are not firmly in the socket in the uterus, they don't always grow together like they should. My daughter had to wear a Velcro® body brace — we called it the "paratrooper outfit" — for about eight weeks. After that, she never had hip problems again. In the end, it wasn't a big deal; but needless to say, I was freaked out about it at first and would have liked to have known this was common for breech babies.

Hut, Hut, Hike! (Vaginal Births)

As I mentioned, both my kids were born via C-section, so this section was written based on interviews with friends and family members who have had vaginal deliveries. That said, I didn't know I was having a C-section until the day before my first baby was due, so I felt like a ticking time bomb, waiting to go into labor at any moment, wondering: Where will I be? Who will help me? How am I going to get myself to a hospital if I am on my own and in labor? The answer… you won't know, but it will all work out. Here are some highlights of the vaginal birth process.

Going into Labor

You are in labor once you start having contractions, but that doesn't mean the arrival of the baby is imminent (in most cases). What it feels like physically to be in labor depends on the woman. For some, it feels like back pain, and for others strong menstrual cramps.

I was taught in my labor classes that first-time moms could typically take their time getting to the hospital because labor can take many hours. Of course, there's always the exception, but most doctors suggest staying at home until you are closer to delivery. You'll be much more comfortable at home than at the hospital (unless you are in significant pain — then, the hospital may be the place to be because they can give you drugs). Be sure to check with your physician about when you should call the doctor (i.e., your water breaks; frequency of contractions) and/or when you should head to the hospital.

In any event, most women tend to start their mental clock for "being in labor" once they check into the hospital.

Water, Water Everywhere

For most women, your water won't break until you are well into labor. But it can happen earlier. A friend whose water broke went to the hospital and they put her on Pitocin to get her contractions going. However, it is my understanding that most women typically experience at least some contractions before their water breaks.

Some women feel or even hear a pop when their water breaks. If your water does break, I'm told it feels like you have peed on yourself. The amount of liquid varies, but you would definitely notice it.

And it is not always a gush of water. Some women spring a small leak rather than a dam break. If this happens it may feel like having a constant urge to pee. And how is that different than any other day of your third trimester? You likely will experience contractions as well, or it will be harder to control what you think is your bladder because it is actually a leak. If you aren't sure, call your doctor.

Lastly, sometimes when you are in labor at the hospital, the doctor will break your water to make your labor progress. It is done with a hook and just feels like a lot of pressure.

Checking In to the Hospital

Your contractions will increase in frequency and intensity as your labor progresses. If you check in to the hospital pretty early, typically your contractions are manageable at that point.

After you're checked in, you are given a room. Once there, you can put your things down and get comfy in the hospital-issued gown. You should use the restroom once you get to your room because they will hook you up to monitors and it may be a while before you get to use a restroom again.

Note: Had I gotten to this point of the process, I would also be trying to go #2 for fear of birthing a baby and a log in front of my husband and a team of people stationed at my vagina. But, truthfully, though this is a common worry, it's not that big of a deal; you have so much going on down there during delivery you won't even notice, and your nurse will be ready with a wipe so discreet and lightning-quick no one else will really notice, either.

Continuing on. The nurses hook you up to monitors that measure your contractions and monitor the baby's heartbeat. Depending on your situation, you may not be continually monitored, but if you get an epidural, most hospitals will continually monitor you. Generally, you will also get an IV for fluids and any necessary medications (like Pitocin if you are being induced). You may also get a catheter, which is removed, before you start pushing.

Being Induced

If your doctor wants to induce you, try not to stress too much about it. Talk to your doctor about why he or she wants to do it (common reasons are being way past due or stalled labor). Just think of the bright side, scheduling (or jump-starting) your delivery removes the ticking time-bomb factor. Plus, you can get all your ducks in a row. If you are a type-A person, this is a really good thing. Just keep in mind that induction might affect your birth plan. Pitocin® increases the pain of contractions, which might make you want an epidural. But that's okay, because if you need Pitocin®, it is you and your baby's best friend.

Just Say No?

A lot of people have a lot of opinions about whether or not you should have an epidural when you deliver your baby. There is a ton of information out there. Read it and then make a decision that is right for you. As the daughter of a pharmacist, I have always had a healthy respect for modern medicine. Not to mention, I am a total weenie when it comes to tolerating pain.

Yes. I'll Have... the Epidural. Right Now... Please and Thank You.

During a typical vaginal delivery, once you have reached a certain point in your labor, you can get an epidural. (Cue the choir of angels!) If you need an epidural — if the pain is too great or you are too exhausted to be effective in labor — it feels like nothing short of a miracle.

If you are being induced, I am told you can request the epidural at the same time, however, that can slow down your labor. (A description of the epidural process is located in the previous C-section section.)

Doing Hard Labor

For a large portion of the labor, you and your partner are together with frequent visits from the medical staff. Whether you let anyone else in the room is up to you. Some doctors cap the number. As for me, I couldn't imagine having people looking at me during labor. In fact, it's probably a good thing I ended up having C-sections. As I mentioned, I don't handle pain well, and I am pretty sure I would have been a total shrew to my husband during contractions... but, I digress.

Walking can be helpful during labor. This is when you are glad you have your robe and slippers. This is also when your own music can be quite soothing. Personally, I imagine I would forever associate whatever songs I heard with labor.

You might expect that the doctor and nurses are with you while you are in labor, but this is typically not the case. The doctor checks on you regularly when you are in labor, but you will be mainly attended to by nurses until you start pushing.

Pushing

The nurses and doctors will let you know when it is time to push. Often a nurse and your spouse each hold a leg and the doctor or midwife is there to "catch" the baby. Some women push for hours, while other women just push only a few times. Brace yourself — they are going to tell you to push like you are having a bowel movement (lovely, huh?). It feels like doing sit-ups while holding weights on your chest to make it extra hard.

A friend told me that when you are pushing during a vaginal birth and you have an epidural, you can't tell if you are really pushing because you can't feel it. She said you just make a funny face and hope that what you are pushing out is a baby (and not a turd).

One mom I know (who did not use any drugs) said that walking was not an option for her because the labor pain was so crippling. Also, when she was pushing, the labor pains actually subsided, so she was really focused on pushing the baby out.

Drum Roll, Please ... Your Baby Is Born!

Congratulations, you are a Mommy! Once your baby is out, the doctor will hold up your child for you to see and the umbilical cord is cut.

It varies from hospital to hospital, but the nurse will usually wipe the baby off and hand him or her naked to you so you can cuddle skin to skin. Keep the baby close to your chest, covered, so he or she doesn't get too cold. After a few minutes of bonding, the nurse will take your baby to a station in the room where he or she will be cleaned up more thoroughly. This is when your spouse, already overprotective and worried about the baby's eyes, will take a ton of pictures without the flash. (By the way, they put a greasy ointment in newborns' eyes. I was told it is an antibiotic that prevents blindness.) Anyway, the nurse will attach a security tag and an ankle bracelet with an ID number that matches your wristband. Next, they dress your child in a diaper, t-shirt, and cap before swaddling the baby in a blanket.

While all this is happening, your doctor will help you deliver the placenta. They ask you to push, and sometimes a nurse will push on your stomach to help it along. If you have an epidural, it's just like the rest of the birthing — you don't really feel it. If you have a tear, you will be stitched up once the placenta is out. There's so much going on, you may not even notice this happening.

Now for the good part — your baby (now clean and swaddled like a giant burrito) will be placed in your arms. Congratulations, Mom!

If you are planning to nurse, now's the time to get started. It's a lovely bonding moment for you and your little one, and the sooner you get started, the sooner your milk will come in.

It is absolutely surreal when they put your baby in your arms for the first time. I remember having to wait for my babies. After each C-section, I had to go to the recovery room without my baby. I think it was about an hour, but whatever it was, it felt eternal. This is one of those things I wish I had known up front, so it's definitely something to ask about if you are having a C-section. I was torn between sentiments like "Don't be mixing my kid up with somebody else's, I'm not sure I could even pick him out of a lineup yet!" and "Wow, my belly is much bigger than I thought it would be now that the baby's out. I feel like Santa."

But really, when they bring you your baby who is on the outside of you instead of on the inside of you, it's really incredible to hold them. It's weird to look at your baby and realize you don't even know them yet. Pretty much all you want to do is look them over. You want to lay eyes on that tiny foot that has been playing soccer with your spleen in utero. But since baby is all bundled up and warm, you wait to do that until later (or I did anyway).

A friend of mine said she was given good advice during her first pregnancy: Sometimes when you hold your baby for the first time, you are giddy with adoration and love. Sometimes you are scared. Sometimes you are overwhelmed. Sometimes just exhausted. It's all normal. It's all OK.

Fun With Your Postpartum Body

Rrrrrip! (When Your Baby Has Ripped You a New One)

When and if it happens, you won't feel it if you have an epi-dural. Now, that's a good argument to take advantage of modern medicine if I've ever heard one! Some doctors will perform an epi-siotomy (when they purposefully cut you in advance), but most of my friends said their doctors didn't do them because they believe you heal faster if you tear naturally. There are degrees of tearing: 1st – 4th degrees, with 4th being the worst.

If you have a tear, it will hurt to sit upright. You will be given ice packs to put on your private area.

Another thing you can do to alleviate the pain of a tear is to take a sitz bath. Basically, you sit in a tub of water that fits on your toilet seat and it flushes water through your stitches and cleans and soothes the area. As much as it hurts at first, it feels better afterwards. The hospital will also supply you with a little bottle you use to gently squirt water into your sore undercarriage for a few days.

You can also use witch hazel-infused or medicated pads. You place them where your tear is and it reduces itching and swelling. (Yes, your tear will itch quite a bit when it is healing.)

Tip

☆ *A hospital nurse showed a friend of mine how to make a fantastic homemade ice pack. Tear open the top of a newborn diaper and fill it with crushed ice. Then use the sticky tabs to close up the "ice pack." My friend said her husband made several of these for her a day and referred to them as "glorious."*

Like a Water Balloon, but Less Fun

Your uterus is still expanded for a few days after birth, not to mention filled with fluid and blood. Your stomach will feel like a water balloon, a bizarre sensation that is compounded by your tired and disjointed stomach muscles. Give it time; it will pass.

The Period from Hell and Praying to the Poop Gods

Let's talk about the mesh panties. After you have a baby (C-section or vaginal) you get a period like you wouldn't believe. Since you can't get up right away, you get to wear an adult diaper in a pair of net panties. The nurses change you regularly, which is humbling, but just part of it. Every time they put your baby in your arms, you don't really care.

Also, when you are in the hospital after you have your baby, a nurse will come by periodically to check the location and firmness of your fundus (the top of your uterus). The nurse will massage the fundus, which causes it to tighten and contract. The massage is unpleasant, but necessary. The nurse may even show you how to locate and massage it yourself. Your uterus will continue to shrink over the next few weeks, especially during breastfeeding, and may feel like contractions or strong menstrual cramps.

Your period continues when you get home from the hospital. You might pass some clots, and if you see anything that looks big, call your doctor and talk with them about it. I had a friend who was passing multiple large clots and had no idea that was not normal.

Now, I would be remiss if I didn't tell you the most painful part about having a baby (even a C-section) is actually the first poop. It will be agony if you don't take your stool softeners like clockwork until you heal up a bit. Additionally, it is common for the first poop to take a few days to arrive. You've been on liquids and the drugs they use to induce and numb you can lead to constipation.

So, I have a story for you, but I want to preface it with the fact that this is not part of every new mom's experience. Out of all my friends who have had babies, this is the only friend I know of who had a pooptastic challenge of this magnitude. But I want to share it with you because: 1) it's funny; and 2) it could happen.

My friend waited about three days to start taking her stool softeners after the birth of her second child. As a result, she did not poop for TWELVE days! She endured several days of ineffective, self-administered enemas and suppositories. When she was telling me about it, she said, "There's nothing like having your husband walk in on you, lying naked on the bathroom floor, atop a trash bag, giving yourself an enema."

Ultimately, she ended up in the emergency room for something called "manual disimpaction."

"I prayed for a doctor with small hands," she said. "Thankfully, he took pity on me and ordered a hospital-grade enema," she continued. "It is not an overstatement to tell you they pumped a gallon of what looked like Italian salad dressing up my ass and then I shit all over the floor. That's right, ALL OVER THE FLOOR! I'm having flashbacks just thinking about it," she concluded.

In summary, stool softener is your friend. Heed this warning, or writhe in pain as you pray to the Poop Gods.

Making the Most of your Stay at the ~~Hilton~~® Hospital

So, you have had your baby and your loved ones are anxiously waiting to see your little one. Each new mom and dad will want to handle the receiving of guests differently, but I will warn you that it can be overwhelming to have a large group descend on you at once.

I strongly recommend you take your visitors in smaller groups, especially if they are bringing their noisy and dirty carrier monkeys — I mean, their kids. Doctors and nurses will come in periodically and need your attention. You will want to hear what the medical personnel are telling you, and if your family is making all kinds of noise, you will be perturbed. It can be helpful for you and your spouse to establish a "get-these-people-out-of-here" code word or signal in advance. Or better yet, share that code with your nurse so he or she can be the heavy.

Remember, you are there to have a baby, not host a party.

Nurses will come and get your baby periodically for various tests or maybe a shot. Also, at some point, your pediatrician will give your baby a checkup in the hospital and come talk to you.

And at some point, someone will come by to take your baby's picture. Hopefully you will love your pictures. Our hospital pictures of our first child were not great, but we thought we should buy them. I think we spent close to one hundred dollars to get enough to send with the birth announcements. Not the best decision, but we weren't really thinking clearly.

We were advised to send our baby to the nursery at night so we could sleep. We did this with our first child, and I still remember an overly cheerful nurse turning on some seriously bright lights at about 3:00 a.m. with my crying baby in tow. It was time for a feeding. I think she said something along the lines of, "Welcome to parenthood!"

My second child was born in another hospital that did not want you to send the baby to the nursery at night. I definitely got less sleep, but I didn't mind.

Lastly, when you are dealing with the gravity of childbirth and on the hormone rollercoaster ride of your life, it is really common to get overwhelmed and have a meltdown. So don't be surprised if it happens to you. Uncontrollable crying is totally normal.

Raiding Your Hospital Cart

When you are in the hospital for the delivery, there is a bassinet on wheels that the nurses and doctors use to transport your baby. In it are baby supplies for your use (diapers, wipes, blankets, etc). Use it; you are paying for it. And don't forget to raid the cart before you leave the hospital.

The hospital receiving blankets are fantastic. They have already been washed many times so they are really soft, and for whatever reason they swaddled much better than the ones we had at home. We totally took a couple of those, but my friend who worked as an OB nurse later told me you are not supposed to do that. So, if I had it to do again I ~~would maybe just take one~~ wouldn't do it.

There also are T-shirts in the cart. Don't worry about raiding those, but just note they are there for your use. You are supposed to change your baby's shirt. We didn't realize this until we were leaving. So our poor kid was in the same shirt the entire four days unless a nurse changed it. That's just one of those things that happens to a firstborn. By the second kid, you know better.

If you are planning to use formula, that's another great thing to raid from your cart before you leave, if it's available. We even asked for a little extra and one of the nurses brought us some. Additionally, the nipples in the cart that go with the ready-made formula actually worked well on a couple of other bottles we had. We liked them a lot, and wished we had taken a few more of those with us.

I also liked the aspirator that was in our hospital cart, although Little Noses® makes a good one as well.

One note of caution on raiding your cart: It's technically frowned upon by hospital staff, so it's probably not a great idea to raid it periodically so they will replenish the supplies. But you should definitely take whatever diapers and formula is left when it's time to check out. There's also a bowl, brush and other grooming items that you are welcomed to take, too. If you aren't sure, ask a nurse.

Tip

☆ Nurses are there to help care for you and your baby. However, do not call for a nurse to come change your baby's diaper unless you are physically unable to do it. That's not their job, that's your significant other's new job when they are in the hospital with you.

Paperwork, Paperwork: Getting the
Birth Certificate and Social Security Card

When you check into the hospital, you get a packet, which includes information on how to order copies of the birth certificate and Social Security card. You will receive an uncertified birth certificate at the hospital; ask your nurse if your state will mail the official birth certificate to you. If not, ask where you need to pick it up (usually city hall), and when.

If it's a big hospital, there may be an office within the hospital where you can submit your paperwork in person before you head home.

Tip

☆ Order more than one copy of the birth certificate, so you can keep them in different places and always have a backup.

CHAPTER SIX

Newborns

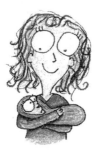

Are You Sure I'm Qualified to Take This Baby Home?

I don't care how many books you've read or how much you babysat. Every new mom has a moment of panic when it's time to leave the hospital and she questions whether or not she knows enough to keep her baby alive. They are so tiny, and dependent on you and your mommy skills. Whatever confidence you built up beforehand is seriously rocked by the gravity of being in that moment. At the same time, it feels like that moment when the rollercoaster starts to glide away from the launching station and you realize… there's no getting off now!

My goal was to do everything textbook-perfect once I got home with baby #1. I wrote down every single thing that happened, and essentially had one eye on my baby and the other on the clock for a couple of days straight because I didn't want to miss a feeding or not be aware of a pee or poop that hadn't happened.

Fortunately, after a couple of days, I started to relax and settle into a groove. You will, too.

Newborn babies sleep a lot — almost all day and night at first. I think this is by design, to give new moms the time they need to freak out and then get used to their new role. All this self-doubt also kick-starts the new mommy boot-camp initiation: exhaustion!

Sleep Deprivation: Laugh, Cry and Bicker

There is so much anxiety those first few nights at home with the baby that you won't sleep well until you pass out from exhaustion. We kept our newborns in the Pack-'n-Play® in our room for several weeks. When your little booger is wide-awake in the middle of the night for no apparent reason, you will learn what's really on TV at 3:00 a.m. By the time you know the jingles and chants for the current infomercials, your baby should be about ready to graduate to sleeping more during the night. And when the time comes to move your baby out of your room, you will feel unbelievably liberated (or I did, anyway).

Words cannot express how tired you will be as a new parent. It's like a fog that impairs your motor and cognitive skills. And it makes you cranky — very, very cranky.

It is advisable now to add a warning. Sleep deprivation combined with learning to be a parent leads to bickering. Every once in a while I would wake up with a vague memory of calling my husband an asshole sometime during our sleepless night. That's not normal for us, but then again prolonged sleep deprivation will affect your behavior in ways you never imagined. Fortunately, it's only temporary.

Eat, Sleep and Poop:
The Importance of Getting on a Schedule

One of the first things you learn from the nurses in the hospital is to feed your baby every three or so hours. Unfortunately, it takes a while for both you and your baby to get on a good sched ule. Your baby has to learn how to eat, go to sleep and poop. You have to learn how to manage all these things and encourage a schedule!

You get to learn this in conditions of insecurity and extreme sleep deprivation. (Lucky you!) But you are not alone — although sometimes you may feel like it — and eventually, you will be on a schedule that works for both you and your baby.

Typically, it takes several weeks for your baby to settle into a sleep schedule. There are some really great books on sleep if you need them. One book that I bought is called *Healthy Sleep Habits, Happy Child*, by Marc Weissbluth.

The following is antithetical to reason, but what I learned from this book is the earlier you put your child to bed, the longer your child will sleep. I used to try to keep my baby up late thinking she would sleep through the night or sleep later the next day. What happened is that she became over-tired and actually slept less!

So I learned to put my child to bed around 8:00 p.m. and if I thought she wouldn't get through the night without food, I gave her a bottle before I went to bed around 11:00 p.m. And then she slept until 7:00 or 7:30 a.m.

There's another book that covers sleep and schedules. It is called *On Becoming Baby Wise,* by Gary Ezzo and Robert Bucknam. (Some people dislike this book because the schedule it suggests doesn't work with their baby, but we modified it based on the needs of our babies and worked for us.) The information really helped me understand how to get my babies to learn to fall asleep on their own. And that, girls, is key!

Tip

☆ *When you are trying to get your baby on a schedule by following a book, remember it's just a guide. There are no absolutes and there is no one-size-fits-all approach to anything when it comes to babies. Through trial and error, you should modify a book's proposed schedule to whatever works for you and your baby. And if what you are trying is just not working, chuck it and find another plan. Call your mom friends or your pediatrician and ask for advice until you find something that works.*

Schedules, when it comes to people, don't remain the same forever, and one of the hardest things for new moms to do is manage the schedule as it changes. For example, at some point your child will sleep five hours instead of three. Instead of thanking your lucky stars and relaxing, you will likely be anxious for hours four and five of that stretch worried about your baby. Why is my baby sleeping so long? The baby should wake up and want to eat. Is my baby OK? I better get a mirror and put it under my baby's nose.

What's wrong?

Nothing. The schedule is changing and you have to change with it. Thank your lucky stars and don't wake that baby! Check on the baby just to make sure everything is okay and then go put your feet up. But, be aware your baby will be extra hungry when he or she wakes up!

Tip

⭐ *My babies always seemed to sleep better with socks on their feet, so after bath time we would put socks on them under their pajamas to keep their little toes warm at night.*

Sharing the Load

The division of labor (well, after the baby is born) is critical to getting into a routine that works for everyone.

If you haven't noticed this with your own mom, one thing you will learn as a new one is that Mom does most of the work when it comes to babies and children — and Mom comes last. Somehow everyone is fed and changed and cleaned-up-after before you even think about sitting down or going to pee. Human nature and what we learn from our parents and other moms train us to put all others first. Thus, you will be joining the legions of other moms who eat cold food that is supposed to be hot.

You can make this better or worse for yourself by the patterns you establish with your spouse when it comes to sharing the load.

For whatever reason, a man and a woman looking at the same space see two very different things. Men see a room. Women see dishes, laundry, dust, a baby to be cared for and things to be put away. This can make the division of labor a bit of a challenge. Just accept the fact that it will probably never occur to your husband on his own to take care of these things. This is one of the many reasons it is a good idea to establish some sort of daily routine where each parent is responsible for certain tasks.

If you are nursing your child every few hours, nighttime feeding is all you. That's why I recommend you abdicate nighttime diaper-changing responsibilities to share the load (pun intended) with your spouse. In fact, I have one friend whose philosophy on sharing the load with her spouse was "I do input, you do output!"

Once bottles were in the mix for us, we alternated the night shift. Even when I was on maternity leave and my husband was working, we still shared nighttime baby duties. Sure, he's going to be tired at work, but he will be with adults. I'm going to be tired at home with the baby. Don't underestimate the importance of preserving your sanity!

When you are home all day caring for your baby, the first thing you want to do when your spouse gets home is hand over the baby. We did this pretty much every day. This was fine with my husband because he was ready for baby time (and I was ready for a break). Sometimes I even needed to get out of the house for a few minutes. So he would take care of our baby while I made a run to the grocery store or picked up some dinner so I could get some fresh air and recharge.

And while we usually handled bath time together (because that is a two-person job for inexperienced parents), my husband took charge of the baby's bedtime ritual each night to help balance the workload.

After all, if you don't share the load, someone other than the baby might be crying.

Babies Cry...

Okay, when your baby cries they are trying to tell you something. (No, it is not "Mommy, you suck!" But you might begin to wonder this as you struggle to figure out what your baby wants.)

What the crying means is: your baby is hungry, has gas, a dirty diaper or is tired. If you have been through all the obvious things and your baby is still fussing and it is 4:00 p.m. and you haven't showered… put your child in a safe place and take an extra quick shower. You will be rejuvenated and better equipped to soothe your fussy baby.

If there is a gas issue in play, I have a bunch of friends who swear by Mylecon®. They use it before feedings and it serves them (err, baby) well. More information on this in Chapter Nine's "Common Illnesses and Tips for Managing Them."

If baby is still crying, try using a swing or bouncy seat with a vibrate feature. And if you are going crazy, put baby in a safe place and walk away for a minute to collect your cool. And you can always ask a friend to come over and help. Everyone has moments, and everyone needs help sometimes, so don't be afraid to ask for it.

And so it goes. You're absolutely exhausted, but eventually you figure it out.

And even if you have no more experience with a newborn than he does, your spouse will always defer to your instincts and look to you for instructions. When your child is crying and your husband is on duty, he'll pretty much do whatever you tell him to do. To that I say… well, the baby is crying because she wants you to fix that leaky faucet in the bathroom!

The Poop Report

As mentioned in the "Original List That Started it All," you will obsess about your newborn's pee and poop. You and your husband will have entire conversations about it as if it was the weather and not think a thing about it. And, in general, after you have a baby, your tolerance for gross bodily stuff increases.

Case in point: Typically, the baby's first poop happens within 24 hours after birth. A black, tar-like poop called meconium oozes out of your baby's rectum. And if you happen to catch it live, it's like watching a slow-erupting volcano.

While no one wants to change dirty diapers, you want your baby to poop. Dirty diapers indicate your baby's digestive system is doing what it is supposed to do. So, you'll be just waiting for that little face to turn red as they grunt. It's kind of weird to rejoice over poo, but, typically, we all earn our first parenting badges the same way.

My husband and I even tracked our daughter's movements on a grid. I made a spreadsheet (my mother is a bookkeeper, which explains this type-A behavior). The record-keeping didn't last very long, but I still have the original "log" — sorry, couldn't resist.

Tips

⭐ *If you have a boy, cover his little wiener with a washcloth when you are changing his diaper; cold air makes them urinate.*

⭐ *Make sure the pooping is over before you change the diaper. I can't tell you how many times I got it all taken care of only to learn baby wasn't quite finished yet.*

⭐ *The color of your baby's poop is an indication of how their little body is functioning. There are even infant poo color charts online that will show you a range of healthy bowel movement colors.*

It's likely your baby won't poop with any kind of regularity at first, which is why it is so important to track it. But if your little pooper hasn't made you a "doodie" in a couple of days, your duty is to check with your pediatrician.

Little Wieners

It's a ... boy! (But, wait — that's not the kind of plumbing I have!) Here's what you need to know about having a boy. First and foremost, boys love their mommies like you can't even imagine. Your son will look at you like you are the sun and the moon, and you will melt and want to give him the keys to your car and your credit card. There really aren't words to express the connection between a mother and son. It will floor you.

Now, about that little wiener... you'll need to decide whether or not to have your son circumcised. Going back to the plumbing I don't have, I totally threw this wiener grenade over to my husband.

Lots of people go for it, lots of people don't. We went for it and the surgery was done by our pediatrician. It was very quick and we were told our son didn't utter a peep! That was our experience, and it was a good one.

After a circumcision, the penis will be a little red around the base. You put petroleum jelly on it and top it with some square gauze that you cup over the penis when you diaper him. You only have to do that for a few days while it heals. The reason you do it is so the wound won't stick to the diaper as it is healing.

Once it has healed, you need to keep an eye on the skin around the base of the penis so it won't attach to the shaft of the penis. Your pediatrician should talk to you in detail about this, and if they don't, ask. (It's not that big of a deal, but it is worth mentioning here.)

Oh, and while we are on the subject of little wieners, I would be remiss if I didn't mention baby boys sometimes wake up with little "woodies." So don't be caught off guard if you get the occasional morning salute!

A Raisin for a Belly Button

The umbilical cord looks like a nasty old raisin as it dries up and eventually falls off. It usually falls off 10-14 days or so after the baby is born (though it can take as long as 21 days). We didn't put anything on the umbilical cord as it was drying up, but we were really careful when giving baths and were mindful of clothing that might affect it. For example, we avoided baby clothing with an elastic waistband. Stick to one-piece outfits at first.

Tip

⭐ *To keep a diaper away from a healing umbilical cord, you can fold the front edge of the diaper under before attaching the closures.*

I have to tell you that we had a bad experience with our first child and the umbilical cord. (I totally snarl and grow fangs when I think about this.) As I mentioned earlier, my first child had some temporary hip problems. As a result, we had to take her to the hospital for a sonogram when she was less than two weeks old. The radiologist doing the sonogram was trying to hold her in this awkward position and actually ripped her little umbilical cord off in the process! She winced and howled, and it bled. Eventually it healed, but accident or not, I still hate that man to this day.

Rubber Ducky, You're the One (Bath Time)

Hopefully, you will get some instructions from a professional on how to bathe your baby before you leave the hospital. We were not so fortunate. We thought our daughter hated having a bath because she cried. She cried because Mommy and Daddy didn't know what the heck they were doing. Eventually, we figured it out through trial and error (poor kid).

Here are a few things we learned:

○ Newborns don't need a bath every day.

○ Typically, until the umbilical cord falls off, you just give your child a sponge bath (and don't get the umbilical cord wet).

○ This is a two-person job at first. Your newborn just lies there like a lump, so it's helpful for one person to hold the baby and another to wash (and take pictures).

How To Give Your Newborn a Bath

Get your supplies together first. You need a baby bathtub, soap, washcloths, at least one baby towel, lotion, a clean diaper, clean clothes or pajamas, a hat (or hooded towel to keep the head warm afterwards) and the camera.

Put the baby bathtub on the kitchen or bathroom counter. It's easier than reaching over to it in the bathtub, and in this location it's still near a water source. Wrap the baby in a bath towel and set baby in the baby bathtub. Cold air makes them wiz, and this isn't your bath, so place a washcloth over baby's privates. It's best to keep them – and their pee source! – covered.

Keeping the baby mostly wrapped up in a towel, just pull out the body part that is being washed. Once you've done so, put it back under the towel as this will help keep your baby warm over-all. We always kept a hat nearby to put on our daughter after we washed her hair. (Okay, head. We had a very bald baby.)

Once their umbilical cords healed, we bathed our babies by sub-merging them partway in the baby bathtub. When you do this you will want to fill the tub with a few inches of comfortably warm water before you put your baby in there.

Tips

⭐ *If possible, position the baby bath tub so that the drain is over the sink opening, so when you are done, all you have to do is open the plug and the water runs right down the drain.*

⭐ *Use a little cup to pour water over your baby's tummy occasionally to help keep them warm dur-ing the bath. And, if it's chilly, and you can do so safely, consider using a space heater.*

Later, when our babies were able to sit up on their own, we

gave them baths in the kitchen sink. (If you do that, just make sure it's clean.)

A lot of samples of baby wash make their way to you through various channels. Baby soap is generally head-to-toe, or all-over soap. If after a bath you notice any changes in your baby's skin, try a different soap. Post-bath, we used baby lotion, but not baby powder, because, as I mentioned earlier, experts say talc-based baby powder can be harmful if inhaled by the baby.

Well, those are the basics. Babies smell great naturally, but a baby who has just had a bath is extra snuggly! They often sleep really well after a bath, too. So keep that in mind as you think about the bath and how it fits into your schedule.

Tips

⭐ *You may be surprised to discover that soured spit-up collects in the folds of your baby's neck. This "baby cheese" needs to be cleaned. When you are washing, gently lift your baby's head so you can get into those folds to clean. After the bath, make sure you dry thoroughly in there. And if the deepest crevices are red and irritated, a thin layer of zinc-based diaper rash cream will help clear it up. It's not a bad habit to get into checking the neck folds every time you change a diaper; keeping the folds clean and dry will prevent irritation.*

⭐ *I liked using two baby towels at bath time. When it was time to take my baby out of the water, I would drape a towel over each of my shoulders, overlapping them on my chest. When I removed my baby from the tub, I would lay her on my chest on the towels. Then I would lift the towel off of each shoulder to wrap it around her and carry her to a place where I could get her dressed.*

CHAPTER SEVEN

Breastfeeding, Formula and Baby Food

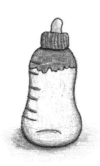

A lot of people have a lot of opinions about whether or not you should breastfeed your baby. I was absolutely amazed at how many people provide unsolicited advice and commentary on something that is really none of their business. And, as I mentioned earlier, people believe they have the right to judge you for your decision, and they will.

Know that going in.

I'm not about to go through the how-to's of nursing your baby (there are plenty of books already dedicated to that topic). However, there are a few extra pieces of information that I found helpful, and I hope you will too.

"Shards of Glass"

I was raised on formula, like many babies from my generation, and I am a healthy and happy person. That said, after reading about the merits of breastfeeding, I decided to give it a try.

Fortunately, I have a friend who talked with me about nursing before my first child was born. She said three very memorable words to me: "shards of glass."

Wow, was she ever right. The first time I nursed (or, rather, attempted to), I could do nothing but throw my head back and mouth the words "… shards of glass." Yeouch! Did it ever hurt!

But I persevered. I found it took a while for the colostrum, and then ultimately the milk, to come in. (Colostrum is a pre-milk substance full of antibodies and other good stuff for your baby.)

I also discovered that even if the hospital provides a lot of support in terms of teaching nursing moms breastfeeding techniques, the medical staff might treat you like a … piece of meat. I remember a nurse that came to do one of my checkups who walked right up to me and without warning poked me a couple of times in the right breast, saying, "Your milk com'n in yet?" I was so caught off-guard that I went into polite mode and simply shook my head "no" while inwardly I evaluated what had just happened. Did she really just poke me in the boobie?

And don't be surprised if a nurse or lactation consultant who is helping you grabs your boob and puts it in your baby's mouth. Try not to be shy, though; there is nothing worse than doing it wrong. And believe me, breastfeeding is a learning process for both you and your baby that takes time.

Uh, You Gave My Breastfed Baby Formula?

It took a while for my milk to come in, so the nurse told me that since my daughter had lost some weight, the hospital had to give her some formula.

The news devastated me. I felt like a failure as a mother, was worried my daughter would have nipple confusion, and I was really pissed that they did it and then told me about it after the fact.

Keep in mind, I was a raging ball of hormones, and this contributed to my stress level.

Had I been thinking rationally, I would have realized it was the opinion of medical people that my baby needed some food and that's why they gave it to her.

And, for the record, we didn't experience any problems from our breastfed baby having the formula.

La-La-La-Lanolin!

The breaking-in-your-boobs part of nursing can lead to severely chapped and scabbed nipples. Lanolin to the rescue! This is the greatest stuff ever. It is thick yellow goo you can put on your nipples that is safe for your baby, and will help you heal as you toughen up.

I didn't have to use it long. In fact, it only took me a couple of weeks to get through the physical difficulties of learning to nurse.

Tips

⭐ *If one side is extra sore from nursing, give the breast a break by pumping that side.*

⭐ *Consider using nipple shields (a nipple shield is a plastic cover with holes at the tip) if your baby is an aggressive eater and you have sore nipples. I have a friend who would use them for a few minutes each time she nursed for the first couple of weeks. Once her baby was partially fed (and not so aggressive), she would remove the shields and finish nursing without them.*

⭐ *When the line of skin underneath your baby's tongue is longer than normal it's referred to as being "tongue-tied." If your baby has difficulty latching, ask your pediatrician or a lactation consultant to check your baby's tongue.*

If you are committed to nursing but experiencing difficulties, focus on getting to the four-week mark. Once you get to that point, it becomes much easier, or it did for me. And if breastfeeding just isn't working out or it just isn't for you, formula is wonderful. (More information on formula is located later in this chapter.)

Showtime, Dolly!

The more you nurse, the more milk your body will make. So, if you feed your baby and then pump, the message to your body is make more milk. Be aware of the messages you send to your body, as it takes time and repetition to regulate your milk supply.

And … if you thought your boobs couldn't get any bigger, wait until your milk comes in. My boobs were unrecognizable. For all you girls who have envied a woman who was more endowed than you, take heart! They pay the fee when it's breastfeeding time. My boobs were so heavy that if they were not in a bra, the sheer weight of them would make them leak. (Oh, and by the way, when you take a shower, the warm water will make your breasts leak right onto your feet.)

Fortunately, your boobs will calm down once the factory finds its groove after a few weeks. Mine went down quite a bit even though the milk was flowing still.

And while it is common for nursing moms to have a dominant boob and a slacker boob, try not to favor one breast over the other, even if your baby has a preference. Your body is listening to those messages, too, and you don't want to end up with a significantly larger breast. Make sure to nurse your baby (and/or pump) for the same amount of time on each breast.

Tips

☆ *Hydrate if you are nursing. Drinking lots of water helps keep the milk flowing.*

☆ *Things change so double check with your nurse or lactation consultant on this, but I was told at the hospital that breast milk was good for four hours on the counter, four days in the refrigerator and four months in the freezer.*

☆ *Sometimes babies will cluster feed (need more food during a period of time). If you are a nursing mom and have stored extra milk, this is an excellent time to rob the milk you banked in the freezer.*

☆ *If you skip or postpone a feeding, make sure you pump to avoid engorgement (pain in the breast caused by unexpressed milk) or mastitis (infection of the breast).*

Another thing that a friend warned me about is that when you first start to nurse, your body knows that the baby is out, and your uterus will contract. This was particularly helpful to me as I had a C-section and didn't have a clue what a contraction felt like. (It feels like a strong menstrual cramp.) I only noticed it a time or two when I first started nursing.

Now, here's something people told me that I was hoping would be true: "Breastfeeding will melt the fat right off your postpartum body!"

Fat chance! It may work that way for some people, but I had a different experience. When I was nursing, my body actually bulked up. My upper arms and back got bigger. I presume this happened so I could carry around the "factory." All (okay, most) of this went away though when I stopped nursing.

Pumping

Checking out a breast pump for the first time can be more than a little intimidating. There are so many parts and pieces and tubes that you may be confused about how this octopus of a contraption actually works. So, here's the skinny.

Basically, a breast pump is a machine that sucks air. You attach a bottle to a breast shield (a cone-looking thing that fits on your boob) and a long skinny tube connects that to the pump.

When you turn on the pump, it sucks air at repeated intervals, mimicking the sucking that a baby normally does. A drop of milk will emerge on the tip of your nipple and then another until it pools into a drop and falls down into the bottle attached to the breast shield. (Eventually, it will become a stream or two of milk, but you have to work up to that.)

Start on the lowest level and increase the strength of the suction gradually. Warning! Do not underestimate the boob-sucking power of a breast pump! If you turn it on too high, you will cry and try to rip it off, but you can't. You have to break the suction of the cone on your breast with your fingertip to get it off — much like you do with a suction cup on the shower wall. So, do yourself a favor and start slow.

Some people love pumping, some people hate it, and some people only pump and bottle-feed. It's different for everyone.

I will say that breastfeeding is very convenient. If you are breastfeeding, a lot of times there's no need to make a bottle, because you are the bottle. However, sometimes you need to use a bottle with your baby. Perhaps your spouse wants to feed the baby, or you have scheduled some much-needed freedom and you won't be able to nurse, or you are going back to work. What do you do? Get your handy-dandy pump and take care of it!

Tips

☆ *If you breast pump regularly, you may find your milk production is inconsistent from day to day. If so, freeze the surplus from the extra-productive days so you'll have enough for the low-flow days.*

☆ *The timing of when to pump is critical. Your baby will need to eat, and your boobs will be the alarm clock that determines when you have to be back to feed your baby or to a place where you can pump again.*

☆ *If you are not at home and need to pump, the car can be a good option, provided you have a power source for your pump.*

☆ *If your car doesn't have an outlet plug, consider buying a car adaptor for your pump. They don't cost much, and they are very handy.*

While there is some gear to contend with when you pump, you might find that pumping and bottle-feeding is a lot faster than nursing your infant. Babies get all warm and go to their happy place and fall asleep a lot when you are nursing them.

Tip

⭐ *If your baby is falling asleep when nursing, try tickling baby's feet to keep them awake. And if that doesn't work, try taking off their clothes. Even though it seems counterintuitive to want to keep a baby awake, it's worth it; they'll sleep better with a full tummy.*

In contrast, a breast pump is steady and gets the job done without hesitation. Another thing I really appreciated about pumping was you knew exactly how many ounces of milk your baby would get because you could measure it.

And once you are done, you can relax knowing that someone else can take the bottle and see to your baby's needs.

Mastitis

A couple of my friends who were nursing moms experienced mastitis (infection of the breast). Typically it starts with sharp pains in the breast, and eventually the breast gets hard and has red streaks all over it. One friend was able to manage it with regular warm compresses and a heating pad for a few days. Another friend had a fever of 103 degrees and said when she nursed it felt like needles. "I had never heard of it and was quite freaked out," she said. "I called the OB and they said it happens all the time. I got an antibiotic and slept all day. My husband had to take a day off of work to take care of us, and then I was fine," she continued. One thing she mentioned to me is that it does not affect the milk, "So it's okay to keep nursing, but it hurts like hell!" While she never knew what caused it, she says she would have loved to have known about mastitis BEFORE the red streaks, fever and rock-boobs, which is why I am sharing this with you.

A Formula for Success

Breastfeeding is amazing for many reasons, but one thing I didn't like about it was feeling tethered to my child. That, and also that when it was time to get up in the middle of the night, it was all me.

My maternity leave came and went. I returned to work only to be relocated by my employer from Washington, D.C. to Atlanta, Georgia. So, while most new moms stress about going back to work across town, I had to get on a plane and go to another state for a week at a time until we could sell our home and move. It was only for a few weeks, but it was cruel, and I still twitch when I think about it.

Ultimately, the move was great for us, but it presented a challenge when it came to nursing. I didn't have a lot of extra milk stored in the freezer, so we were forced to introduce formula.

I didn't know it at the time, but this would be one of the most liberating experiences of my new mommy life. My baby didn't miss a beat, and I really felt okay about it.

The downside? Formula does affect baby's poop. It makes it smellier. The upside? Formula gets it done. Whether you breastfeed in addition to that or not, formula is wonderful (expensive, but wonderful).

Tip

☆ *This is worth repeating: A just-fed baby is like a can of soda, if you move them around a lot, they explode. To reduce spit up, try to keep your baby somewhat still, with head slightly elevated, after a feeding. This is also good if your baby has reflux.*

As I mentioned earlier, people will judge you for using formula. But I still don't understand why other people think they get a say in what's best for you and your baby. The important thing is to find something that works for you, and there is nothing wrong with formula. Using it doesn't mean you love your baby any less. A happy mommy is the key to a happy baby. And formula-fed babies are healthy, too.

The Joy of Rice Cereal
and Pureed Meat in a Jar

When your baby is four to six months old, your doctor will tell you it is time to start feeding your baby solid food. They typically recommend that you start with rice cereal and try other foods one at a time, so if your child has an allergic reaction it's easier to identify what food caused it.

Our doctor gave us a whole list of Stage I fruits and veggies to give to our daughter. Which of them do you choose first? We weren't sure, so we applied logic. We thought it would be better to start with veggies so she wouldn't get hooked on the sweet ones. So we started with green beans. Looking back now, I realize that was brutal because they taste as gross as they smell! My second child benefited from this mistake as we started with applesauce.

Tip

☆ *Beware of bananas. They can cause constipation and shouldn't be up first on the list of foods to give your baby.*

Rice cereal can change the consistency of your baby's poop, and cause constipation. It can also affect their sleep habits; babies sometimes sleep for longer stretches once they start eating baby food. (More on constipation in Chapter Nine in the section called "Common Illnesses and Tips for Managing Them.")

CHAPTER EIGHT

Going Places With a Baby

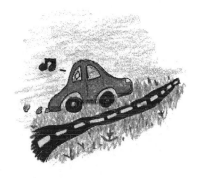

Getting Out the Door

Most pediatricians recommend you keep your baby out of public places for about the first six weeks to minimize their exposure to germy people. Can you say, "cabin fever?!"

When it's time, you will start venturing out on your own with your baby. It can be a little intimidating at first to take your baby somewhere by yourself. After all, in your home environment, all your gear is close at hand. When you leave, you have to determine what you will need and balance that with what you can carry or fit in a stroller.

At first, it's hard to know what to take, so you'll pack it all just in case. That's normal. When your car looks like that of The Beverly Hillbillies™, you know you are a new mommy venturing out with your newborn for the first time.

It takes a while to master the art of getting out the door. Not only do you have to dress your unrecognizable body, but you have to prep your baby as well. Just to be safe, plan an extra 15-30 minutes to get your baby and gear together. If you're meeting up with someone else, you might as well start working on your "sorry-I'm-so-late" spiel. No matter how organized you are, your baby will see your keys in your hand and spontaneously poop or spew vomit. That's just how it goes. Eventually, though, you can get out the door with less effort.

Tip

☆ *An indoor shopping mall is a good destination if you are going out alone with your baby for the first time. It's climate-controlled and you can walk to several places without having to load and unload your baby into the car.*

Take the stroller and carry the things you need in the storage compartment underneath. If your infant carrier doesn't close up, bring a blanket to cover it to keep people from touching your baby.

Well-meaning people will ask to see your baby. When this happened to me, I obliged them, but always positioned myself in the way to keep them from getting too close. Maybe that was rude, but I didn't know where the person had been or what they had touched.

Most people use common sense and won't reach into the baby carrier, but then again the world is full of idiots. Be prepared to speak up or show them your "uh-don't-touch-my-baby" expression to stop them if it's necessary. It's more important to protect your newborn from germs than to be polite to a ~~moron~~ well-meaning stranger.

What Goes In the Diaper Bag?

So, what's in the bag? (The diaper bag, that is.) Here's a list to get you started. The rest you figure out as you go.

☐ **Diapers**
Pack one diaper per hour to be safe

☐ **Wipes**

☐ **Bottles/Baby Food**

☐ **Clothes**
At least one change of baby clothes. (If you don't take this, you are just asking for it!) You might even want to throw in an extra T-shirt for you on the off chance there is a poop explosion.

☐ **Blanket**

☐ **Changing Pad**
Keeping one of these handy will ensure you'll have a clean changing surface any place you need one. You

can buy disposable changing pads or just use a folded-up or just use a folded up receiving blanket. If I was using a changing station in a public restroom, I would put paper towels down before I put my changing pad down. Those changing tables are probably very germy and my changing pad is going to go back into my diaper bag with all of my baby's things.

☐ **Disposable Plastic Bags**
For dirty diapers or poopy clothes.

☐ **Toy**

☐ **Pacifiers**
Note this is plural.

☐ **Tether/Pacifier Cover/Teething Gel**

☐ **Burp Cloth/Cloth Diaper/Wash Cloth**

☐ **Infant Tylenol®**

☐ **Hat/Mittens**
(If relevant)

☐ **Hand Sanitizer** for you and **Sanitizing Wipes** for surfaces your baby may touch

Tip

 Put diapers, wipes and pacifiers in your car and other places you frequent. You never know when they will come in handy.

CHAPTER NINE

Baby Wellness

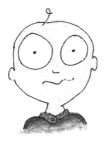

Medical Must-Haves and Resources

It's easy to get overwhelmed by all the stuff you can buy for your baby. While there are lots of things that can help you along the way, there are a few medical "must-haves" in my opinion. Here's a list:

- ☑ Infant Tylenol® and Infant Ibuprofen®
- ☑ Thermometers (ear or temporal, and rectal)
- ☑ Aspirator (a booger-sucker)
- ☑ Infant Saline Drops (nose drops)
- ☑ Cool Mist Humidifier

Tip

☆ *Talk to your pediatrician at each checkup about the proper kind and dosage of pain reliever/fever reducer for your baby's weight, and write it on the box. The dosage changes as your baby grows.*

It's also important to know how to find your own answers when it comes to questions about your little peanut. Here are some resources to keep in mind.

The Nurse Line

Most pediatricians have an after-hours line for parents. It's a good idea to program the number to the doctor's office and the after-hours nurse line into your phone. It's especially handy if your baby is sick during the night not to have to go searching for the numbers you need.

Online Medical Resources

We use the Internet a lot to research symptoms. One pretty good resource is the Health Information section of the Mayo Clinic web site. One note of caution: Take everything you read on the Internet with a grain of salt. You can easily freak yourself out trying to diagnose your baby based on something you've read online.

Other Moms

Obviously, the best medical advice comes from your doctor, but other moms with young children can be extremely helpful to you when your baby is sick. More than likely, they have been through it at some point and can offer some wisdom. They may have taken their child to the doctor and can share with you what their doctor told them. Or they can tell you what kinds of things helped their baby. We moms will try just about anything to make our sick babies feel better, so it makes sense to seek wisdom from other moms, too.

Blogs

Blogs are another place you can find information on pretty much any topic under the sun. There is great value in moms sharing their experiences with one another. Finding a blogger who has kids the same age as yours can be fun because you likely will relate to many of the things they write about. Additionally, I know there are a lot of moms who have kids with special needs that connect and share information through blogs.

Well Visits

When you are at the hospital and your pediatrician comes to see you, they tell you when to schedule your baby's first checkup.

When you bring your baby to the first well visit, don't make rookie mistake #1: taking your newborn into a room with sick kids. Generally, a pediatric office has separate waiting areas, one for sick patients and one for well patients. If your baby is well and you are just there for a checkup, enter with your baby into the well-child waiting area.

People in a waiting room are idle and therefore might be interested in passing the time by taking a look at your baby. Even in the well-waiting area other children will look like germ-infested carrier monkeys. Sometimes they can't help but try to touch your baby. Adults are no better; total strangers will touch your baby's head and, worse, hands! Don't forget to remove the temptation by closing the shield or putting a blanket over the baby carrier.

Tip

 If a child wants to touch your baby, you can oblige them by letting them touch your baby's feet.

A well visit typically includes a weigh-in. You take your baby wearing only a diaper to the scale, but then they'll ask you to put your child on the scale without a diaper. If that diaper is soiled, you'll need another one to put on your baby. Keep one nearby.

Before you leave the pediatrician's office, typically they schedule your next well visit. The recommended well-visit schedule according to the National Institutes of Health, through age two as of this writing is as follows:

◎ 1 month	◎ 6 months	◎ 15 months
◎ 2 months	◎ 9 months	◎ 18 months
◎ 4 months	◎ 1 year	◎ 2 years

All practices are different, but typically you make well-visit appointments with your primary pediatrician. If your baby gets sick and needs to be seen by a doctor, you may only get your regular pediatrician if he or she is taking sick visits that day. In practices with several doctors, they rotate such duties.

Tips

⭐ *If you are on your own at the doctor visit and there's a lot of walking involved, make it easy on yourself and put the infant carrier in the stroller.*

⭐ *Consider the appointment time carefully. You will be exhausted and sleep-deprived. Maybe you don't want the first appointment of the day. Or, if the practice is a particularly busy one, maybe the first appointment of the day means you can get in and out more quickly because there isn't a line of people in front of you waiting for the doctor.*

⭐ *Additionally, Mondays are often a bad day to do well visits because kids who get sick during the weekend are at the doctor on Mondays, which can cause delays.*

Immunizations

There are quite a few vaccination shots at first. Shots are the worst. There is always this moment of silence from your baby's indrawn breath. Silence … silence … red face … open mouth … and finally, the wail! You will feel like dirt, but that's normal.

Okay, so here's my take on immunizations. The shots are intended to keep your child healthy. I kept track of the shots that my baby was due for, and read about them in advance so I was informed. The Mayo Clinic web site has a list of the recommended vaccines by age and what they protect against.

There is a lot of debate about them, so you need to do your homework. My husband and I did all the required shots for our children and experienced no problems. However, we didn't always do them the way the doctor offered them. For example, if multiple shots were required, we broke them up by making additional appointments and paying additional co-pays. We felt better about avoiding a cocktail of immunizations in our baby at one time.

A note of warning: on more than one occasion, I encountered a nurse who made it clear she thought I was silly for doing this. To that I write, screw her! She doesn't know (or care) about what's best for my baby. That's my job.

And it's yours. **You** decide what's best for your baby.

Tips

⭐ *If your child is scheduled for a shot, be ready with a pacifier (if they will take one) to help soothe them.*

⭐ *A friend told me that she would give her baby Tylenol® before a scheduled shot. If you have Tylenol® in your diaper bag, you could always ask your pediatrician if they think your baby will need it. Some shots are more painful than others.*

Common Illnesses and Tips for Managing Them

Again, I am no doctor, so consult with a medical professional if you think your child is sick. Here are a few things to be aware of:

Congestion

Unless you live in a plastic bubble, at some point your baby will become congested. Saline nose drops and an aspirator (a.k.a. a booger-sucker) are your friends. This combination does wonders. Actually, if the baby can hold their head up, I have found that nose drops followed by tummy time is very effective. This is mostly because kids hate it and infant pouting in the form of huffing-and-puffing tends to work some of that mucus free (and then gravity does the rest). If your child is older or particularly strong, be advised you might need help holding down your bucking bronco while you suck boogers and they cry. If you hate the fact that they start to cry — realize that crying may help break up the congestion, too.

Tips

★ *If your baby is congested, sometimes it helps to elevate their head when they are sleeping. Using a bouncy seat or swing will achieve this. Another option is to elevate one side of the crib mattress by putting a folded or rolled up towel underneath one side of the mattress. Obviously, you don't want it to be too high, or your baby will just end up sliding down. I know some moms who did this for babies with reflux, which is when baby has a hard time keeping food down.*

★ *A friend of mine suggests getting in a steamy shower with them to help relieve congestion. If you don't want to juggle a wet wiggly baby in the shower in the middle of the night, turn the shower on its hottest setting, put a comfy chair or blanket on the bathroom floor, and snuggle your sickie in the steamy room.*

One time, I thought my son had chest congestion (rather than nasal congestion), but was told babies' torsos are so thin that congestion in the nose can be felt in the rib cage. If you feel rattling in the chest area though, I'd still take your baby to get checked. Better safe than sorry.

Constipation/Gas

If rice cereal or other baby foods cause constipation in your child, your doctor may recommend giving your baby an ounce of water in a bottle. If that doesn't work, your doctor might suggest giving apple-prune juice (diluted 50/50 with water) as a next step. For example, half an ounce of water mixed with half an ounce of apple-prune juice was helpful for our baby. Another option is to give your infant baby food prunes. Warning! Tread lightly with the prunes — they can send you directly into a poop-up-the-back situation.

Tips

☆ *If your baby is constipated, your pediatrician may recommend you use a rectal thermometer to stimulate a poop. To do this, put a disposable plastic sleeve on the thermometer, add a dab of lubricant on the end, and insert just the tip in the bum for a few seconds — just like you would if you were taking the baby's temperature. Sounds gross, I know, but that's what our pediatrician advised, and it totally worked.*

☆ *Another thing you can do for a gassy or constipated baby is to try taking her legs and bending the knees up and gently pushing them toward the belly. Also, you can gently rub your hand in a clockwise motion on the lower belly. My pediatrician told me this is the direction that the intestines process food.*

Croup

When you hear barking coming from your baby's room, it might be a viral infection of the vocal cords, voice box and windpipe called croup. No one tells you about croup, but most kids get it at some point before the age of six, and it usually manifests in the middle of the night – lucky you!

You will know your baby has croup because they will have a very distinctive cough. It sounds like a barking seal. Sometimes your baby's breathing is labored, too. It is really scary for new (or even experienced) parents, especially if it is your first encounter with it.

Call your doctor. If it's the middle of the night, and you are awaiting a callback from a doctor or nurse, you should turn on your humidifier and sit close to it with your baby. If you don't have one, you can go into the bathroom and turn on a hot shower to make steam and sit in the bathroom with your child. Conversely, cold air also helps. If it's cool outside, you can bundle them up and take them out into the night air, or you can also open the freezer door on your refrigerator and let them breath the cool air from the freezer.

Tip

⭐ *If your little one is uneasy, sometimes it helps to distract your child with a book or a toy while you sit by the humidifier or in the bathroom.*

Reflux

All babies spit up, but reflux is when babies regurgitate a fair amount of breast milk or formula. If there is a significant amount of spit up (or vomit) several times a day, or your baby is coughing a lot after each feeding, you should talk with your pediatrician about reflux. Another indication of reflux might be if your child arches their back and cries after feedings. Some babies just can't handle a large volume of food. If they eat too much the food is sent back up the esophagus, which can be painful.

My friend who had a baby with reflux said that the doctor put her infant on formula for sensitive tummies and prescribed a mild reflux medication. Note: The amount of reflux medicine you give your baby will increase as your baby gains weight, so you may be in the pediatrician's office every three to four weeks for a weigh-in so the dosage can be adjusted.

After about six months on the medication, my friend and her husband were able to stop using the medicine (it's worth noting that they initiated that change). Their daughter was fine; she could eat and drink whatever she wanted without problems.

My friend's advice for new moms dealing with reflux is as follows: "You have to find a schedule and food or anything else that helps your baby. You also have to ignore a lot of advice about letting them cry it out, not rocking your baby to sleep or holding your baby too much because you will spoil them, etc."

Tips

☆ *If your child has reflux, try to keep your baby still and upright for at least 20 minutes after feedings. Some babies need to be held longer.*

☆ *Smaller, more frequent feedings can also help your baby keep food down. Your doctor may also suggest adding some rice cereal to a bottle to help the baby keep the food down.*

☆ *Using a pacifier just after a feeding can also help babies with reflux.*

Colic

We didn't experience colic, but the same friend who dealt with reflux did. She said one of her babies cried a lot and needed to be held at a certain time every evening. It started when she was two months old and lasted two months. Her baby cried and was extremely fussy from 7:00 p.m. to 10:00 p.m. To soothe her, my friend walked around with her for long periods of time. The rest of the time, she said she was a very happy and smiley baby.

Tip

⭐ *To help soothe a colicky baby, try swaddling your baby tightly and bounce them up and down. My friend said she would bounce lightly on an exercise ball while playing a CD that had a washing machine sound on it. She got the CD at Babies "R" Us® and raved about it.*

Eczema

Some babies have eczema (thick patches of dry skin). My son had it, and it was particularly itchy for him in the winter, but otherwise didn't bother him too much. I had been putting lotion on it, but it was still there. So, at my son's regular checkup, I asked his doctor about it. She said to put cortisone cream on it three times a day for three days to see if that would clear it up. Basically, this was presented to me as an alternative to lotion. It didn't occur to me to ask the doctor more questions about the cream.

I happened to mention this to my dad, who is a pharmacist. He informed me that cortisone cream is, in fact, a steroid. Huh, what? My doctor didn't mention it was a steroid. I also learned from my father that if it's used too frequently, it could affect a baby's bone development. He said it should be used sparingly.

Although ultimately my father and I do not think any harm would have come to my son from using the cortisone cream for a period of just three days (as the doctor advised), I decided that, instead of using it, I would try different lotions for eczema that I got at the drugstore.

I also talked to other moms, and, eventually, I found one that worked better for my son. It's called Aquaphor®, and we used it after his bath and other times as needed.

While we're on the topic of eczema, when I asked the doctor about it, the immediate response was to medicate (use the cortisone cream). Perhaps what I should have done was ask what causes eczema. From a mom friend I learned there are food triggers for eczema, so I looked them up online and then paid attention to those foods in my son's diet. Sure enough, certain foods trigger my son's eczema. Once we eliminated those foods, his eczema improved.

Tips

★ Ask lots of questions about what a doctor is recommending (even if it's something that seems as straight forward as topical skin cream). You should also ask questions about what causes the problem and other alternatives they sometimes recommend.

★ Then go online and talk to your mom friends about it. You can't be too informed.

★ Remember, I am not a doctor.

Teething

Yes, I know teething is not an illness. But it can make you think your baby is sick. Um, why is that?

Teething (which begins when your baby is only a few months old) can cause fevers, runny noses, irritability and sometimes diarrhea. Why no one told me this, I have no idea. But it's something to keep in mind if your baby is at teething age and having any of these symptoms.

Since we're talking about teething, I must mention we used a product called Baby Orajel Teething Swabs® on both of our children. These look similar to standard cotton swabs, but there is numbing medicine in the stem. When you bend it in the middle, the medicine moves to the tips of the swabs and you can use it (rather than your finger) to apply numbing gel to your baby's sore gums. I also liked it because you are only numbing a tiny area. As with any medicine, there are some people who suggest you shouldn't use it, but we did and found it helpful.

Tips

★ During one of your doctor visits, be sure to ask about using Tylenol® and Ibuprofen®. If baby is teething or sick, and you are using this medicine regularly to combat a fever, you may need to alternate medicines to avoid having too much of any one medicine in your baby's system.

★ Other tips for teething include giving your child a cool wet washcloth to chew on and providing a liquid-filled teething ring that has been cooled in the refrigerator.

Use Your Instincts

Be an advocate for your child's wellness. You are the voice of your child. It is up to you to process information from doctors and decide what it means for your child.

You know your baby and the situation better than the doctor. You have instincts about your baby — even if you don't know what the problem is or how to fix it. If you sense that what the doctor is telling you does not jibe, speak up! It's all you. Your baby can't talk, so you have to ask questions and more questions, and do your own research. Seek another opinion if something doesn't seem right.

Doctors are fantastic resources. You have gone to a lot of trouble to select one who is right for your family. You should depend on doctors for good counsel, but here's the thing: You could ask several pediatricians the same question and get several different responses. What one doctor says is not always the gospel. You have instincts for a reason; pay attention to them.

CHAPTER TEN

New Mommy Wellness

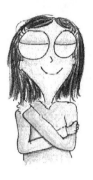

Your Brain

Hormones: Yelling at Strangers and Crying Over Toothpaste

Hell hath no fury like that of a post-partum mommy. My second pregnancy was very different from my first. I'm not sure if it was because I was having a boy instead of a girl, but I was unbelievably aggressive. There was almost no filter on my mouth at home or at work. No topic was off-limits, and no one was immune from my occasionally rude and scathing remarks. Sometimes I would catch myself in one of those out-of-body moments and apologize immediately after I had done or said something a little too direct. But most of the time, I really didn't care. At the time, I worked in corporate America and fully believed it was time for a little truth-telling at the old office. In fact, my super sarcastic friend at work really got a kick out of it and even began referring to me as "Mean Heather." Luckily, my fire-breathing phase didn't jeopardize my job while I was pregnant. Fortunately, people cut me quite a bit of slack.

Fast forward to the birth. Things were going great. Everything around me was as it should be. I was feeling pretty good. And then came the hormones. A few weeks after the birth, my husband took us through the drive-through at a fast-food restaurant. As we waited (forever) to move along the drive-through line, a car cut in front of us in line.

[Raging hormones enter stage right.]

I got out of the car and stood in front of the offending vehicle. I flailed my arms and yelled at the driver. There was a kid in the front seat, so I did not use any obscenities, but there was no mistaking my message. The driver very wisely decided to ease out of the drive-through line, which made me (and my whacked-out hormones) very happy.

And the best part of it all was my husband's face. His sweet little wife had just shocked the hell out of him. Behold the power of female hormones!

Things settled down for a while, but when my son was about eight months old, I hit another snag. I had some little crying fits, but mostly I was just PISSED OFF! My sunny disposition had become a Class V hurricane; I was not myself, and my poor husband had no way to check the weather forecast.

I hated, I mean HATED, everyone at work (except my close friends). Everything seemed like a conspiracy to piss me off. I was out of control. I had this recurring fantasy. I would quit my job in a blaze of foul-mouthed glory pumping my middle fingers up and down giving everyone "the bird" with gusto as I walked backwards out of building with a booming, wicked laugh. Fortunately, I confided in a friend who told me I was depressed and suggested I make an appointment with my gynecologist.

I was so surprised! I had done some crying, but I never thought of depression as rage and severe bitchiness. It was. I was diagnosed with Postpartum Depression (PPD).

I think it's important to point out that this wasn't just following the birth of my child, but several months later. I think that is part of the reason I didn't catch on sooner. The hormonal roller coaster ride lasted a little longer for me than I realized it could; stress, big lifestyle changes and lack of sleep can also really take its toll. So be aware if this happens to you. If you are lucky enough not to get whacked with the PPD stick, excellent! Maybe having read this though, you can help a friend if you spot the signs. Some of the signs are weepiness, an out-of-character increase in cursing (or, in my case, mentally plotting the demise of co-workers too stupid to be on the payroll).

As I mentioned, I had almost no filter on my mouth. In fact, one day at the lunch table, I turned to my dear friend and co-worker and said, "Do you have to talk that loud? 'Cause you're yell'n in my ear." There was stunned silence at the lunch table. My friends and I still laugh about that incident, but you get my point, right? If you see any of these signs in a friend, send her to her gynecologist and pray she doesn't shoot the messenger!

Help! I think I'm Crazy

When I had my first child, I was plagued with weird dreams. I had really vivid dreams where my baby was in danger and I had to save her. I also had some crazy thoughts about her. What would happen if I (fill-in the-blank)? Then I would freak out wondering why I was thinking this.

After some pondering, I decided it was me reconciling the fact that my tiny little baby was wholly and completely dependent on me (and my husband) for survival. It's pretty heavy stuff.

Don't beat yourself up over crazy dreams or thoughts; they are completely normal. That said, if your thoughts are stronger, very intense or frequent, or you are even a little bit concerned about them, please talk with your spouse or another mom, and call your physician.

Tip

☆ *Having a new baby can be trying. There is a lot of societal pressure to act like you are having fun when you are not. So focus on the positive, but don't feel like you have to act like it's all roses all the time. Most of it is great; but some of it just sucks.*

"Mommy Brain"

You need to know there is something that happens to your mind when you become a new mom. I've heard it called "Mom Brain" or "Mommy Brain." It's sort of like having chronic brain farts. It's basically a more intense version of "Prego Brain." You can't remember things, and it takes you longer to do things. In general, you just feel less sharp. You might even forget the most routine things. It's a phenomenon I have neither explanation nor recommendation for. Just know it can happen and it is just part of Mommyhood.

Now that you're a mom, there are so many additional things you are responsible for — and some of them are huge, as they involve caring for your baby every minute of every day. Not to mention you are sleep deprived and very rarely get time to yourself.

When you are on overload, "Mommy Brain" can make things even harder. One thing that might help is to make a list to help you remember what needs to get done. Personally, I find great satisfaction in crossing things off my to-do list. It's proof I actually managed to accomplish something in my quest to meet the demands of motherhood and beyond!

"Mommy Brain" diminishes in intensity over time — but I still have the occasional brain fart and attribute it to Mommyhood.

Your Body

Fat Pants

Take any delusions you have that you will go home from the hospital in your pre-baby jeans and throw them out the window. Unless you are Heidi Klum, you will still look very pregnant when you leave the hospital   and for at least a couple of weeks afterwards.

For me, a month after my son was born, a very excited first-time mommy-to-be asked me when my baby was due. Naturally, I was devastated (and she was mortified). Amazingly, I went into polite mode and tried to make her feel better for having said something so stupid. I'm not sure what I said, but what I didn't want to say was, "Oh, that's okay, I do still look pregnant!" I had lied to myself that I was looking OK and this was a huge dose of reality.

Remember all that water they pump into you before you give birth? That, plus swelling, plus air bubbles if you have had a C-section, contribute to being bloated for a few weeks.

Now if you are one of those people who, after giving birth, look like you never had a baby, good for you. The following is not for you rare and lucky Heidis (damn you), this is for all the regular women like me. Here it is: the fat-pants rollercoaster is one that nobody wants to ride, but most people can't get off for some time.

My closet was full of all sizes of pants I bought as I slimmed down after my first child. Looking on the bright side, I actually was able to wear many of my fat pants during my second pregnancy, which kept me out of maternity clothes longer.

On the not-so-bright side: the week before you are scheduled to return to work (if you are a working mom), you need to start trying on work pants to find out what will fit. This is traumatic, so be prepared. Whatever lying to yourself you have done will become painfully obvious during this exercise.

After you know what doesn't fit, I recommend a trip to a store with bargains galore to get some inexpensive pants that do fit. Size doesn't matter in this case; you will look worse in clothes that are too small than in clothes that are a size you never thought you would wear. So, get some fat pants that feel flattering and cut the size tag out.

Also, you will discover that, post-baby, you will experience random periods of weight loss. There are two paths you can take during these times. You can have a piece of pie, or you can take advantage of your momentum and make better choices. Do yourself a favor and eat an apple instead. Your new hiney will thank you when you look in the mirror.

The worst part of all of this is remembering my pre-baby body and all the "problem areas" I thought I had. Oh, how I long for my worst pre-baby fat day! But take heart; if you make good choices over time you can get back to where you once were, or close.

As I mentioned, during my first pregnancy, I gained a whopping seventy pounds – which is a lot for someone who is 5'4" with a small frame. I was ultra-passive about getting it off, and it took nearly two years.

During my second pregnancy, I only gained forty pounds and I was a lot better off for it. Then, after giving birth — and despite working a full-time job and having two young children, I made time to walk a few times per week with my neighbor. I graduated from my fat pants at a much faster rate, and then I could make the ceremonial walk down the hall to take yet another pair of too-big pants to the guest room closet. (Sometimes, I even heard Pomp and Circumstance in my head as I walked.)

Fighting the Battle of the Bulge

Okay, so some unwanted cellulite has taken up residence on your body. To get beyond it, start holding yourself accountable for what you are doing today.

Get on a food plan — whatever kind of plan works for you. And get on an exercise plan — whatever kind of exercise plan works for you. Do you have a friend or a neighbor with whom you can walk? Do you have a pal who is in the same boat who can help keep you on track with your exercise? If you have access to a gym, use it. Just dedicate the time. Plus, it's a built-in break from everything else in your revised life and it will give you time to think. If you don't have access to a gym, no problem! You can get online and look up exercises where you just leverage your own body weight. Or go to the library and get a book. I really like *YOU: On a Diet*, by Mehmet C. Oz, MD, and Michael F. Roizen, MD.

I can tell you from experience that if you just wait for it to happen naturally, or think nursing your child will melt that fat right off your body; you will be disappointed. Unless you are really young, after you deliver your baby you get to keep some of the weight you gained during pregnancy as a parting gift (great).

Yes, you can get it off, but you have to do a little work to help things along. And unless it will motivate you, stay away from those meat-market gyms where the women look all skinny and slutty (damn them!). I prefer the local YMCA so I can be on the treadmill next to an octogenarian and feel hip.

Tip

⭐ *Your boobs will change a lot if you nurse. Once you stop nursing, get a professional bra fitting. You go to a department store or a lingerie boutique, and ask a salesperson (female!) for help. They measure you over your current bra and make recommendations. Trust me; it's worth doing.*

Post-Partum Fallout

This would be a good time to mention that exercising, laughing too hard or sneezing after you have a baby can lead to the occasional bladder issue, but usually it's minor.

Another bodily change to be aware of is that some of your hair might fall out. Or rather, mine did. I wasn't balding or anything, but I was sort of alarmed because no one warned me. This usually stops when your hormones level out after a few months.

Speaking of fallout, we should probably talk about hemorrhoids because there are few things you should know that could help you. First, they are very common. Second, medicated pads and creams for hemorrhoids are your friends. And, third, if you have a persistent problem with hemorrhoids, go to the doctor. A friend dealt with visits from "Uncle Roid" for a couple of years before finally going to a specialist. Her doctor scheduled an outpatient procedure that was quick and relatively painless. Obviously, every situation is different, but in this case, she wished she'd taken action sooner.

Tips

☆ *If you are embarrassed to see your general practitioner about it, go see the nurse practitioner who can refer you to a specialist.*

☆ *My friend also shared a tip with me. She said sitting on the Boppie® pillow gave her some relief from her hemorrhoids.*

Um, You Want Sex? But That's How We Got Into This Mess!

So, you are half-crazy and fighting the battle of the bulge in your tagless fat pants. Your boobs are unrecognizable (not in a good way) and you are sleep deprived. You've been through the hormonal ringer and you are not quite yourself. You don't know what you are doing with your baby and your house is a mess. It's been six weeks and your deprived husband wants sex. Really, you want sex? Holy crap, that's how we got into this mess in the first place!

My husband wasn't at my gynecologist follow-up appointment, and that was to my advantage. I'm pretty sure I lied to him about how many weeks I was supposed to wait. Well, the truth is out now! Sorry, honey, it was self-preservation!

Ladies, as my doctor told me, you just have to get back into the swing of things. Remember, he loves you and doesn't care about your totally messed up body. You just have to get back to it!

Note: If you think you can't get pregnant when you are nursing, think again! (Don't forget your contraception.) The other thing that I didn't realize is that the older we get the more eggs we ovulate in each cycle, which increases our probability of having multiples. I learned this from a friend who went for kid number two, and got kids number two and three! Why no one tells you this, I have no idea. So, here's your heads-up, ladies!

CHAPTER ELEVEN

Working 9-5,
Then 5-9

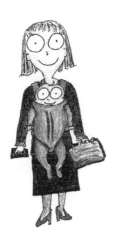

Should I Stay or Should I Go Now (Back to Work)

I f you can choose whether or not to work after you have your baby, stop and take a minute to appreciate that you even have that choice.

Trying to decide? Every mom is different, and sometimes you just don't know how you are going to feel until you have actually held your little peanut in your arms.

Sure, staying home or going back to work is about the kid(s). But if it's not financially required, I believe whether or not you stay home or go back to work depends on what makes you — the mom — happy. Don't worry about what anyone else is doing. You are the one who knows what is best for you. The grass isn't always greener, and there are good things and bad things about each scenario.

Having been a working mom and a stay-at-home mom, I can give you perspective on each situation.

Positive Things About Being Home:

- I get to play with my kids during the day. When I was working, I didn't get very much time with them during the week. I would see them early in the morning and just before bed.

- I know more about how they interact with their friends, respond to new situations and strangers, etc.

- Being home pays dividends in your kid's behavior. When I see a behavior problem, I can correct it the way I want it corrected.

- We all eat better. I have more time to devote to meal planning and meal preparation (yet somehow I still manage to burn dinner once in a while).

◎ I have more time to exercise and take care of myself.

◎ On a gorgeous day, I can be at the zoo instead of in some dumb meeting.

◎ I read more. (I need to in order to keep my brain stimulated.)

◎ I take more pictures and have managed to keep them fairly organized.

◎ My kids get more sleep. When I worked, my kids had a later bedtime, so that I could spend more time with them in the evening.

◎ There is less guilt about not being with the kids.

Negative Things About Being Home:

◎ Your identity changes. I didn't realize how much of my identity I associated with my job. At first, I found myself inserting references to my working days in defense of an ego that still associated success with a paying job.

◎ I actually get fewer things done. I'm always really busy, but accomplish very little that is identifiable.

◎ Living on one income instead of two is a huge adjustment, so there is more finance-related stress. I didn't realize how much I took disposable income for granted. I totally miss my paycheck and going out to lunch (and the shoe store) with my work friends.

◎ My house is messier. It is a constant struggle to keep it clean because we are always in it messing it up.

◎ Our grocery bill is much higher. When I was working and the kids were in childcare, meals were included. Thus, our food bill was substantially lower. (Technically, it was wrapped up in other expenses, but when you are evaluating your budget and you remove the childcare bill, you need to add money to the food category).

◎ We also go through a lot of paper goods. This is directly related to the messing up of the house and the eating (and later, the pooping) at home. I try to be as earth-friendly as I can, but I can't live without my paper towels.

◎ Sometimes I feel like I have lost my edge mentally, like I am not as sharp as I was when I was working.

◎ I definitely look less put together. My clothes are much more casual. I have traded in most of my cute dress shoes for flip-flops and sneakers. It's sort of sad to go into a shoe store now and have no reason to be shopping for cute shoes. Of course I look anyway and always find something I like. Then I ask myself the question, "Where would I wear those? Chuck E. Cheese®'s?" Then I totally buy them anyway and schedule a Girl's Night Out so I can wear them. (On the upside, my mom shoes are rather comfortable.)

Positive Things About Being a Working Mom:

◎ Having a two-career household enables both parents to experience the working and parenting worlds as equally as possible. You can both have careers, participate in childcare and take care of things at home together. You don't have separate realms (but we all know the woman does way more work!).

◎ Not everyone is meant to be a stay-at-home mom. Some moms are happier when they work outside the home. While I absolutely love being home with my kids, in some ways I think I was a better mom when I worked because my life was more balanced. Not only did I feel fulfilled by my career, but the time I spent with my kids was focused, quality time. Also, I liked contributing financially to our family, and we all very much enjoyed the lifestyle that a dual-income situation provided.

⊙ Lastly, if you enjoy your career, you will bring that confidence and excitement home with you.

Tip

☆ *If you need to make a change, look for the type of job that suits your growing family's needs. There are plenty of employers who support flexible work schedules that allow moms to volunteer at the school, coach teams and drop-and-run when their child is sick. You could also explore part-time employment at your current job, or look for a new part-time job altogether.*

I know it may be hard to evaluate this kind of decision because you've never been a working mom or a stay-at-home mom. But, remember, at the end of the day, you'll be a better mom if you are happy. Good luck if you're trying to decide. I'm sure you will make the right choice.

How to Stay Home and Stay Sane (or Close Enough)

When I was a desk jockey in Corporate America, I thought staying home with kids would be harder than going to work every day. It totally is. It wasn't something I desired, but staying home is what happened, and I am not sorry about it (most days).

When my daughter was three and my son was almost one, my husband found a job he really wanted in another city, so we moved. I left my career (and paycheck) behind.

Without a doubt, there is an adjustment period. It takes a while to figure out how to do it. That is, how to stay home and stay sane. These are some things that might help:

Find Other Moms

It's great to spend time with moms who have a baby (or kids) the same age as yours, so you have someone to talk with who is probably having similar experiences.

Mother's Day Out

I'm so thankful for Mother's Day Out! A little time to myself is crucial to my ability to remain a stay-at-home mom.

Exercise

Regular exercise is a great stress reliever and it is good for you AND you get a break from your child (assuming your gym has childcare). This is a really important part of my sanity, and it's money well spent in my opinion. Plus, I am not required to go to an office, so really there's no excuse not to exercise.

If you don't belong to a gym, there are plenty of free ways to get exercise. If your kids are with you, put them in a stroller and go for a walk. Or let them amuse themselves around you while you exercise at home. When you go to the store, park far away and hike the few extra steps while schlepping your little beloved and a diaper bag on the way into the store. This pays dividends, as I mention in "Fighting the Battle of the Bulge" in Chapter Ten.

Girls' Night Out

I need my girlfriends (and sometimes a margarita) to be sane. Girls' Night Out is absolutely precious to me. I'm really thankful for my pals for helping me stay sane (or close enough). If your friends aren't calling, call them. They might think you're too busy to take a break (what?!). Let them know you're eager to reconnect.

Quiet Alone Time

Some people recharge with social activity. Others require a lot of alone time. If you do, read, take a bath or do whatever grounds you and makes you a happier person. Pay attention to things that take away from your quiet time (like talking on the phone — although sometimes, that can keep you sane, too). When I get in a car by myself, I don't turn on the radio. I simply enjoy the silence.

Date Night

Your baby becomes the center of your universe. Don't forget your marriage. Arrange the occasional date night and go have some fun with your spouse.

Tips

★ *Some moms treat the name of a good babysitter like a matter of national security. Be advised a mom may not recommend her favorite babysitter to you for fear you will book her on a night she needs to use her. I recommend you seek out people you know and trust to babysit in addition to asking your mom friends for names of sitters.*

★ *If you find a really good one and pay her well, she will usually make time to help you.*

Going Back to Work: A Contrail of Tears

Going back to work is traumatic for any new mom. You have to leave your baby and are still really messed up hormonally. Most women have to go across town, but as I mentioned, I was in the process of being relocated by my company and had to get on a plane and fly away for a week at a time. Having done some research before that first flight, I learned that the airline considers a breast pump a medical device, so I took it as a carry-on item.

On that first airplane trek away from my baby, my pump and I went to the security checkpoint at the airport. The young guy who scanned the pump asked me about it.

I was feeling very emotional and hormonal at the time, not to mention I was a total basket case because I would rather have my eyelids tattooed than fly on an airplane.

At first, I thought he was going to give me a hard time, but then I noticed he flinched when he heard the words "breast pump." Sensing an opportunity for light-hearted self-distraction, I started talking and using those words a lot — loudly emphasizing the word breast over and over again because it clearly made him uncomfortable.

I was thoroughly entertained as he waived me through just to make it stop.

When I landed in Atlanta and got my bags and rental car, I proceeded to my hotel. On the way there, I came to a tollbooth for which I was not prepared. Luckily, I was able to scrounge around and come up with enough change to get through. But when it was my turn to put in the money, I missed the basket and threw the money all over the ground. The evil tollbooth lady was nasty to me and ultimately waved me through with disgust. I guess it was karma for having tormented that poor TSA guy. I cried all the way to my hotel.

Okay, enough about me. Here are some things to know about returning to work:

- ◎ You won't want to. It takes about a month to get back into a groove as far as getting up and out the door.

- ◎ When you are at work, you just go through the motions at first. You will think everything your coworkers are freaking out about is ridiculous and you will say to yourself, "This isn't important! My baby — that's the stuff of life! THAT is what's important!" Remember, though, you are at your job and you can't completely disregard workplace concerns. Just roll your eyes on the inside and go with the flow.

◎ For the first month or so you will hit the baby-craving wall every day. This withdrawal can be addressed by looking at pictures of your baby online or at your desk.

Tip

☆ *When returning to work, think about what will happen when you get the call that your baby is sick. Talk to your employer and your spouse about it ahead of time.*

◎ If you have some flexibility, I suggest you make your first day back a shorter one than normal, like from 9:00 a.m.-3:00 p.m. And if you can, don't make your first day back to work the first day your baby goes to child-care. See if your spouse or a family member can watch the baby that first day. This will alleviate some of the stress you are experiencing.

◎ Try to throw yourself into your work. Concentrating on every task and staying very busy will be good for your away-from-baby stress and your career.

◎ If your child is going to a daycare or someplace outside your home for care while you work, bring over your wipes and diapers and anything you will need to have there in advance. I was hauling my baby and all that crap on day one; it sucked. Live and learn.

◎ Time your arrival at daycare so that you have 15-20 minutes to spend there with your baby. The first day is not the day to drop your child off and run. Bring tissues (and antidepressants!). Also, make sure you have the phone number so you can call later and check in on your child.

Pretty soon, you will do it all without thinking about it, and eventually you won't remember it any other way.

Tips

☆ *The night before go you to work, pack the diaper bag, and, if possible, make bottles and label them. That way you just get them out of the fridge and you are off!*

☆ *Don't forget the pacifier and tether, baby blanket(s) and clothes. My son often came home in a different outfit than I sent him with.*

☆ *If your child is awake when you are getting ready in the mornings, tag-team with your spouse so you can get your showers done. When I was nursing, it was ideal for me to feed the baby before I showered. Then my baby could settle into a happy place while I finished getting ready.*

☆ *Whatever you do, be careful handling the baby once you are in your work wear. I changed many a top before running out the door.*

CHAPTER TWELVE

Super Moms

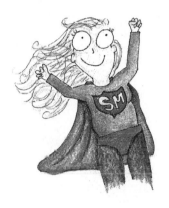

There are lots of super moms in the world, and those are the ones you want to befriend and emulate. You can learn *so* much from these women.

There is a HUGE difference between a mom who is super and a supermom. But, for better or worse, supermoms (or "perfect moms") are going to be part of your motherhood journey. My advice to you when it comes to these women is to be mindful of, and limit your exposure to, the moms that are unhealthy to be around.

There are so many incredible moms out there. If you don't have the right ones around you, keep looking. They're out there, I promise. Finding and hanging on to the right friends will make a big difference in your life as you become a mom.

The Perfect Mom is a Unicorn

Wherever you go, you can always find someone you think is doing it better than you. You can also find people who want to tell or show you that they are doing it better than you.

[Supermoms enter stage right.]

There is really no such thing as the perfect mom, just like there's no such thing as a unicorn. Sure, you can take a horse and put a cone on its head, but that doesn't make it a unicorn.

Yet when it comes to motherhood, there are varying degrees of this charade. Images and stories in movies and books and online can give an unrealistic impression of what "good motherhood" involves. And some women work hard to mirror those images.

The reality is, we are all figuring it out as we go along and we all make mistakes. Despite appearances, no one really has it all together. It's not any easier for the next mom (unless that mom is some super-wealthy famous person, who has an entire staff of people waiting on her family, hand and foot).

I have found the people who work the hardest to show you they have it all together are typically the ones who are the most insecure about how they are doing. They use their perfection facade to feel better about themselves. It helps them to believe they are superior. The sad thing about this is that a mom who is more vulnerable about the challenges of motherhood might actually feel worse after an encounter with a "perfect mom."

Take heart, ladies! Everyone struggles, and everyone questions what and how she is doing. So don't let anybody make you feel like you are a lesser mom. Motherhood comes with real insecurity, but remember what Eleanor Roosevelt said, "No one can make you feel inferior without your consent."

The formula of motherhood is complicated by your personal situation, but when you peel back the layers, I believe all moms are created equal.

Know-it-all Moms:
I Got Your Kryptonite Right Here

It must be a requirement, because everyone has a friend or family member that falls into the category of the know-it-all mom. These are the ones that talk more than listen and are just waiting for an opportunity to tell you: 1) how you're doing it wrong; and 2) how they do it correctly.

Motherhood is a whole new category for the one-uppers of the world. It's highly annoying — especially if you ask another mom a question and she gives you an answer laced with condescension. How are you supposed to know? You're a new mom and that's why you're asking!

Remember that while some moms act like they know everything about kids, the only expert on your kid is you (and your spouse, of course).

I remember talking with another mom who had just had her first baby, too. She confidently dispensed advice to me that I later discovered was completely wrong. So my advice to you is to rejoice and commiserate with other really new moms, but don't put too much stock in their input. Consider their lack of experience in the trenches and choose your mommy confidants wisely.

Okay, are you ready for your kryptonite? Here it is, one simple phrase to say to know-it-all or perfect moms... "Good for YOU!" Be prepared for a hasty exit after that one, but it is a really nice way to respond to someone who is basically putting you down.

Remember, too, that you might be a new mommy now, but eventually you will be in a position to help another new mom. Make mental notes about how other moms talk with you and emulate the ones you admire when it's your turn to pay it forward.

Mom Friends & Other Friends

When you have a baby, you have involuntarily joined a hood — the Mommyhood. The way you see the world changes whether you want it to or not. A hurt or missing child is more horrific to you than it was before. Petty things that used to bother you or matter to you just don't anymore. Your mind and heart are so focused on your baby you can tune out the world around you for large chunks of time.

You come out of the haze when you need some help. After all, mothering this tiny life has just been put squarely upon your shoulders, and you are going to need people to talk with about it. *[Mom friends enter stage right.]*

Hopefully, you have a mommy pal or two with whom you can talk. If not, look for ways to meet other moms. Find a group through online channels or chat up moms you encounter as you go about your daily life. They're everywhere. Look for ones that take a common sense approach to things and don't fall into the know-it-all category. Sometimes it takes trial-and-error to find the right mom or moms to talk to, but you'll find them and you'll learn from them. They are awesome for a lot of reasons. They will teach and advise you. They can give you the skinny on all aspects of motherhood. And while they may hold close the phone number of their favorite babysitter, they will totally listen to your poop story while you share a bowl of bean dip.

Unfortunately, your friends without children likely won't be able to help you with the mom stuff. And sometimes they have a hard time relating to you in your changed state. Depending on the situation, they actually can become a little jealous of you, so be careful with your non-mom friends. Bear in mind the dynamic between you has changed for them, too; they might need some time to adjust to you being a mom first and their friend second.

And note that your non-mom friends shouldn't be replaced by your friends who are moms. In fact, I still spend a lot of time talking to my friends who don't have children (I love them, and) I can reach them. It can be hard to get talk-time with your mom friends because they're so busy.

Additionally, some moms are all-kids-all-the-time. They don't pursue outside interests. If you do, then focusing on those interests can be a great way to remain connected with your friends who don't have children. And remember to stay interested in your single friends' lives. I'm sure they are interested in your little one(s), but will want to talk about what's happening in their world too.

When it comes to birthday parties or other kid-centric events, think carefully about whether or not to invite your friends who don't have children. Unless it's your very best friend who wouldn't miss it for the world, they probably don't really want to come.

Friendships also change when both you and your friends have babies. If you wonder what kind of mom you will be, I can tell you. Generally, I have found that whatever kind of person you are is the kind of mom you are. If you are a sweet and caring person, you will be a sweet and caring mom. If you are a self-absorbed and snotty person... well, your friends will still love you, but they might not hang out with you as much once kids are in the mix. Likewise, you might not be able to overlook character flaws you tolerated in your friends once you see that their apples (who are playing with yours) didn't fall far from the tree. If you have a friend who is raising little hellions, you won't want your kids to pick up their bad habits. But, I digress... this is something that you will be dealing with a little later.

In summary, when it comes to friends, having a baby is like becoming a Girl Scout® where you learn: *Make new friends, but keep the old – one is silver and the other's gold.*

CHAPTER THIRTEEN
Making Memories

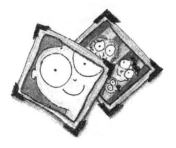

Dear Baby

From pictures and video to scrapbooks and blogs, there are many ways to record events and memories of your kids. But the one that means the most to me is a simple letter.

When my first child was born, my husband and I wrote her a letter when we were in the hospital. The letter detailed the day's events and recorded our thoughts and feelings about her birth. We also wrote about her and what her arrival meant to us. A quick re-read of the letter at any time takes me back. It helps me remember the name of the nurse we liked the best and how excited and sleep-deprived we were. Thanks to the letter, we won't forget, and one day, she will know.

Each year on her birthday, I write her a letter. I include all of the little things about her that she is doing, the words she knows, who her friends are, her favorite toys, and funny things she has done.

The letter doesn't take long, and since I write it just once a year it's easy to do. It is my opportunity to tell her in my own words how grateful I am that she is my daughter.

Of course, I do the same thing for my son now, and we have electronic files for each child with birthday letters in them. I also keep a hard copy in our safe deposit box.

One day, when they are old enough, they will get the letters. And I plan to continue writing to them for the rest of my life.

Picture Time!

Most people take pictures of their babies at regular milestone intervals such as three, six, nine and twelve months, etc.

One of the reminders that your child has achieved a milestone age is the required doctor appointment. Now, here's a rookie mistake I made: I had the morning off of work, so I scheduled the photo on the same day as the doctor's appointment. Good idea, right? Not so much. Odds are your baby will get an immunization shot at the appointment, and that is not the day for a Kodak®

moment. If you want to do the photo on the same day, do it first. A photo session after a shot is just one of the many ways you can have a horrible experience getting professional photos taken Here are some things to be aware of when it comes to taking pictures in a department store photography studio:

- If you can, try to schedule the photo for a weekday, and try to get the first appointment of the day. Many studios aren't great about staying on schedule. And you don't want to be stuck there while the employees try to sell other clients who are in line ahead of you pictures while your child has run out of patience.

- Decide what you want going in so you don't get suckered into a larger purchase than you need.

- Try to time feedings so your baby will be awake and happy. (If your child is cranky every afternoon, don't schedule an afternoon photo session).

- Don't assume the Mensa candidate posing your baby for a picture knows how to handle a baby. If your child can't hold her head up and they want to put your child in some kind of prop that won't work, speak up.

- Be sure to keep your baby calm in the waiting room. When my daughter was around four months old, I took her to a portrait studio at the mall. Even though we had an appointment we had to wait a while for our turn. I passed the time by playing with her. She was so happy and smiley, but when it was finally her turn to be in front of the camera, she was worn out and just looked at us blankly as the photographer and I made fools of ourselves trying to coax a smile.

- Until your baby is older and you really have your act together, bring a backup outfit, but avoid wardrobe changes unless there is poop or vomit involved. You'll probably just have a brief window of time during which your child is cooperative, and you'll want to use that time as wisely as possible.

Organizing Your Photos

If you are like most people, you will take about a million pictures of your baby. Keeping track of all these moments can be hairy if you don't establish a good system.

One really basic way to manage your digital photos is to put them in folders by month. When you download them, just dump them in the current month's folder. After a year has passed, make a folder for the year and put all the monthly folders in that folder. You can also use programs that you buy or download for free to help you organize your digital photos. Ask your friends what they use and look for a system that will work for you.

You will also want to back up your digital photos, so you don't lose them if your computer crashes. I have a subscription to a cloud, which is a digital file backup system. I also upload my favorite photos to a photo sharing and processing site, so I can print the photos I want to frame. That site serves as an additional backup.

Sharing Your Photos

Social media has really changed the way pictures of kids are shared. Just be sure to check the privacy settings. You can't be too careful about who gets access to images and information about your kids.

Which brings us to nudity. It's tempting to share pictures of babies and younger kids naked online, and it's true that little butts are incredibly cute. But keep those photos offline, even if you think your privacy settings are airtight.

One note of etiquette when sharing photos... just pick a few. No one wants to see 192 variations on your favorite pictures of your baby. (Here she is drooling on the pink outfit, and here she is drooling on the blue outfit with the matching bib!) All the pictures will be great to you and your husband — and maybe your mother. But for everyone else, just share a few.

CHAPTER FOURTEEN

Parting Words of Wisdom

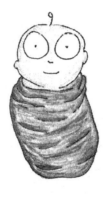

Yes, I'll Have the Baby and Side of Guilt

No one bothers to mention the unbelievable guilt that Mommyhood can bring. All of the decisions that used to be so easy for you now have a whole new dimension...guilt.

As if it's not bad enough that you doubt your new mommy skills, you also have to contend with the guilt that hangs on decisions big and small. From going to the movies with a friend to going back to work, guilt becomes a daily part of your life as you navigate the Mommyhood.

The reality is, when you are brimming with hormones and trying to find out what kind of mom you are, guilt is just something you have to deal with. Constantly.

Try to look for ways to have a balanced life as a mom. For example, you have been cooped up with a newborn for what feels like an eternity. At some point, it's time to go out without your baby. I remember the first time I left my child. Just my mom and I went to Target®. I felt both liberated and horribly guilty. (For crying out loud, it was a trip to Target®!)

Fast-forward a couple more weeks. Now you have been tethered to your new and beloved baby for even longer, and it's time to enjoy some real personal time. Go on a date with your husband or go to the movies with a friend. Or go out by yourself. Check your guilt at the door and just go. You will be better off for having done it.

Going-back-to-work guilt really sucks. To make matters worse, babies start to become really interactive about the time you have to hand them over to someone else. You feel like you are going to miss things. More guilt arrives.

Tip

⭐ *If you are a working mom and feel guilty about it, focus on the swoop — that moment at the end of the day when your baby's face lights up because they see you and you swoop in for the hug. It's a fantastic moment, and one I looked forward to every day.*

Getting It All Done

Getting it all done is not possible. Sometimes you just have to prioritize what you can do and let the stuff that is lower on the list go. Your mantra when you are feeling overwhelmed should be, "I am just one woman." Do your best and reconcile the rest. You can run around trying to be supermom, or you can be realistic, go easy on yourself and focus on being happy.

I promise you your baby will pick up on your cues. If you are frantic and all over the place trying to do all the things you used to do before you had a child, you won't be happy and your kiddo will respond accordingly. So my recommendation is to make happiness your goal.

That said, it takes a while to find your Mommyhood stride. There is plenty of trial and error and that's normal.

A Will of Your Own

You need to make sure you and your spouse are the ones who get to choose what happens to your baby if something happens to you. It should be up to you, so make sure you get your ducks in a row so you get to make that choice.

It's horrible to think that you might not be there for your child, but as a parent, it's something you have to think about. You need to have a will that includes your stated preferences for the care of your child.

It was a really depressing endeavor for us, but I am glad we did it. We hired an attorney that specialized in it and got it done; if you're on a tight budget, free forms are readily available online. We designated three sets of people to care for our children. This allows for our top choices to decline, and covers us (and our children, adequately) should something happen to the designees.

It's really hard to pick someone else to raise your child. After all, no one is you. You have to think about the candidates in a different way than perhaps you did before. You need to consider their philosophies on life, religion, money and education. You need to look at how loving and watchful they are or would be. Would they love your kids as if they were their own? Do you want a person or a couple who already has kids — or not?

Of course, you need someone just like you — but that's not always possible. So then you have to find the person or people among the candidates that are most like you.

We also considered the age of the candidates and their geography. What choice would keep our kids closest to their grandparents? Who would do a good job making sure they see their other family members, and who would make sure they are safe and do their homework when they are old enough to have it? It's really complex, and the more time you dedicate to it, the harder it can seem, but follow your instincts. Make your list, ask your chosen guardians and get it done.

There is peace of mind in having a will of your own.

The Only Thing That Really Matters

There are millions of books, magazines and web sites that cover every facet of parenting out there. They can make you feel pressured to be the perfect mom and raise the perfect child.

You should celebrate and enjoy your baby's milestones. But remember, how early they roll over, stand, walk, talk or potty train doesn't matter at all in the grand scheme of things.

I have found that in the end there is only one thing that really matters. You can give your child every comfort and luxury in the world, but all they really want is you.

Mommy and me classes, baby sign language and the latest and greatest toys are not really what it's about. You don't have to give your child any of these things to be a good mom. All you have to do is be there.

And that, my friends, is the Mommyhood. (As I see it anyway).

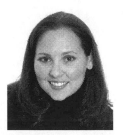

My husband and I have two funny kids who make us snort laugh. We live in Knoxville, Tennessee, where I avoid laundry and write when I can — usually when I am supposed to be sleeping.

I write and curate a blog called TheMommyhood.com, through which I share tips, solutions and humor for moms — basically anything that makes my life easier or makes me laugh. TheMommyhood.com is an upbeat gathering place for anyone who needs a chuckle, so please stop by and chime in. You will be among friends.

And, maybe, just maybe, after a few (rather large) glasses of wine, I might endeavor to finish the book that picks up where this one leaves off. After all, there are quite a few secrets to the toddlerhood.

Connect with me:

Blog: TheMommyhood.com

Facebook: TheMommyhood.com

Twitter: TheMommyhood

Acknowledgements

First and foremost, I must say thank you to my sweet husband who was totally ignored for large stretches of time so I could write this book. And then afterwards he graciously read the manuscript over and over again to help me. Thanks, Bert, you're the best! I wouldn't want to be on this journey with anyone but you.

Which brings me to our kids. When I became a mom, I expected to teach my kids all kinds of things, but the truth is, I have probably learned more than I have taught. Molly and Charlie, you are wonderful people who make me laugh every day. I love you to the moon and the stars and back!

Thanks also to my mom and dad for showing me what it means to be good parents. And to Charlie and Linda who are the best in-laws (like ever). I have watched and learned from you both as well.

To my sisters and to friends who are like sisters to me, thank you so much for your encouragement and support. In particular, I would like to give a HUGE shout out to Angie Pegram Saffoe who happily read every single version of this book despite a very busy job and family life. And many thanks to my friend Gail Yongue for all the time she spent researching medical facts. Thanks also to my friend Jason Rosenberg for always helping me with my pesky legal questions. I am very thankful for all of you guys, and hope you know it.

To my editor, illustrator and dear friend, Heather Hopp-Bruce, thank you for the countless hours of editing and design work you put into this book. I am beyond grateful for your input and contribution, and I thank my lucky stars that I got to work with you on this project. You are the Gary Larson of motherhood, and I encourage anyone reading this to visit www.thebabysucks.com to see more of your work.

And, as for the stories in this book, I must tell you it was Mark Dickens who came running over (all freaked out) to help me get up after I fell down at work because — like an idiot — I was pregnant and wearing heels. Matt Lehigh was the new intern at my husband's office who got the napkins for me when I was flying the barfy skies. Donna Longino was the one who told me I was depressed when I confessed to her that I might involuntarily quit my job in a blaze of foul-mouthed glory. And, last but not least, it was my friend and guru for all things technical, Adam O'Donnell, who withstood me saying in front of a table full of our coworkers, "Do you have to talk that loud, cuz you're yell'n in my ear?!" when I was all hormonal.

I'd also like to acknowledge my grandmother, Ruby Alexander. When I was about sixteen, she gave me a small flowery notebook for Christmas. It was all she could afford to give (and probably more than she could afford to give), so I decided to do something special with it. I used it to record little dreams and things I wanted to do — one on each page of the notebook. When I accomplished something, I would tear out the sheet and mail it to her with a note, telling her what I had done.

"Write a book," as you may have guessed, was listed among the pages. And while I no longer have my grandmother, I am proud to have this page — a page in my first book — I sure wish I could send it to her and tell her all about it.

The Book Club

I want to thank my amazing friends and family members, who read this book in its various forms. And I thank you for allowing me to share some of your stories and best tips. Your feedback was invaluable, and I appreciate your help more than you know. Above all, thank you for being there for me when I needed you.

Carla Arterburn
Whitney Biggs
Heather Hopp-Bruce
Amy Cipriano
Anissa Dalle
Beth Browning-Foshie
Caitlin Hamilton Summie
Victoria Jansma
Jennifer Johnsey
Kirsten Morell
Megan Mullins
Angie Pegram Saffoe
Dana Richardson
Bert Robinson
Linda Robinson
Rachel Samulski
Brooke Templeton
Becky Vollmer
Gail Yongue